Essentials in Stable Angina Pectoris

Juan Carlos Kaski

Essentials in Stable Angina Pectoris

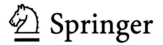 Springer

Juan Carlos Kaski
Cardiovascular & Cell Sciences Res Inst
St George's University of London
London
UK

ISBN 978-3-319-41179-8   ISBN 978-3-319-41180-4   (eBook)
DOI 10.1007/978-3-319-41180-4

Library of Congress Control Number: 2016948438

Printed on acid-free paper

This Springer imprint is published by Springer Nature
The registered company is Springer International Publishing AG Switzerland

This book is dedicated to
My wonderful wife, Marta, for her unconditional love and continued support and inspiration; my father, who is over 90 years of age and still practices medicine with great care and devotion; and to all medical practitioners who strive to improve their knowledge to provide better care for their patients.

Preface

Stable angina pectoris affects a large proportion of individuals in the general population. Recent data indicate that approximately seven million American people suffer from angina. This not only is a very frequent condition but one associated with an increased risk of major cardiovascular events, including myocardial infarction and cardiac death. Chronic stable angina also represents a major financial burden to many individuals affected by the condition and to health services worldwide. Angina is often, but not exclusively, caused by obstructive atherosclerotic coronary artery disease. Coronary atherosclerotic plaques causing progressive stenosis of the arterial lumen can lead to myocardial ischemia as a result of the restriction they impose to coronary blood flow. Coronary stenoses may thus limit the ability of the coronary circulation to meet an increased myocardial oxygen demand. The classical definition of angina based on the above mechanism is, unfortunately, applicable almost exclusively to myocardial ischemia caused by obstructive coronary atherosclerosis. There are, however, many other mechanisms beyond obstructive coronary artery disease that can lead to angina. Indeed, dynamic, functional mechanisms may play a key role in the genesis of angina both in the presence and in the absence of epicardial coronary artery obstructions. Abnormalities of the coronary microcirculation, which have remained elusive to conventional imaging for many years, are now accepted to play a role in "microvascular angina", a condition which is now finally capturing the attention of physicians on both sides of the Atlantic. Microvascular angina is discussed in this book in a specific chapter. The functional aspects of microvascular angina, its clinical presentation and prognosis, as well as the diagnostic tests used for the assessment of microvascular dysfunction are topics discussed in this book. This work also includes clinical diagnostic and therapeutic algorithms, thus trying to bring this topic closer to the practicing cardiologist. A chapter has been devoted to address the different clinical presentations of angina in women and the challenges posed by the many diagnostic and therapeutic differences determined by gender. The rational treatment of angina depends largely on the understanding of the causes and mechanisms leading to angina pectoris in the individual patient. This monographic work presents current treatments as recommended by the International guidelines but also introduces new concepts regarding unmet needs in the management of subgroups of patients with coronary artery disease as well as those affected by microvascular angina. The ultimate aim of this work is to assist the managing physician to identify the different forms of angina pectoris that may come to their attention, all of which pose important diagnostic and therapeutic challenges. In this book I argue that as the current definition (and the understanding) of angina does not necessarily encompass all of the various presentations and pathogenic mechanisms of angina, a change of paradigm is required to serve our patients better.

London, UK   Juan Carlos Kaski

Acknowledgments

I am extremely grateful to Emma Magavern, MD for her help with the formatting of the references and proofreading of the manuscript.

Contents

Chapter 1
Chronic Stable Angina Pectoris: History and Epidemiology

Abstract Stable angina, which affects a large proportion of individuals in the general population, is associated with major cardiovascular events including myocardial infarction and cardiac death, and represents a major financial burden to both the individual affected and the health services worldwide. Stable angina pectoris is characterized by episodes of transient central chest pain, often and reproducibly triggered by exercise, emotion or other forms of stress. The chest pain usually subsides with rest and with the administration of sublingual nitrates. It is established that the anginal pain is triggered by a mismatch between myocardial oxygen demand and myocardial oxygen supply resulting in myocardial ischaemia. Traditionally, stable angina pectoris is considered to be caused by obstructive coronary artery disease. Over the past several decades, however, evidence has accumulated suggesting that vasomotor changes taking place at the site of the epicardial coronary arteries and the coronary microcirculation can also trigger myocardial ischaemia even in the absence of obstructive coronary artery stenosis. This chapter will address issues related to the development of the concept of angina pectoris over centuries and the association of anginal symptoms with both organic and functional mechanisms capable of causing myocardial ischaemia. One of its sections will be devoted to the epidemiology of angina pectoris.

J.C. Kaski, *Essentials in Stable Angina Pectoris*,
DOI 10.1007/978-3-319-41180-4_1,
© Springer International Publishing Switzerland 2016

Introduction

> Angina pectoris has seldom been completely cured yet still we
> must not despair as in time we may arrive at its true cause and
> administer effectual remedies. A. Lawler (Lecture at the Royal
> Medical Society in 1800)

Stable angina pectoris is generally characterized by episodes of transient central chest pain, often and reproducibly triggered by exercise, emotion or other forms of stress. The chest pain usually subsides with rest and with the administration of sublingual nitrates. The anginal pain is triggered by a mismatch between myocardial oxygen demand and myocardial oxygen supply resulting in ischaemia. Traditionally, stable angina pectoris is considered to be caused by obstructive coronary artery disease. Over the past several decades, however, evidence has accumulated suggesting that vasomotor changes taking place at the site of the epicardial coronary arteries and the coronary microcirculation can also trigger myocardial ischaemia even in the absence of obstructive coronary artery stenosis. The development of the concept of angina pectoris over centuries, and the association of anginal symptoms with both organic and functional mechanisms is intriguing. Stable angina affects a large proportion of individuals in the general population, is associated with major cardiovascular events and increased mortality, and represents a major financial burden to the individual and health services worldwide.

History

Descriptions of chest pain associated with heart conditions and death can be found in ancient Egyptian, Greek and Roman writings as cited by Deines et al. [1] (Fig. 1.1) The term "angina" has been reportedly found in writings by the Greek physician Hippocrates (460–370 BC), who believed

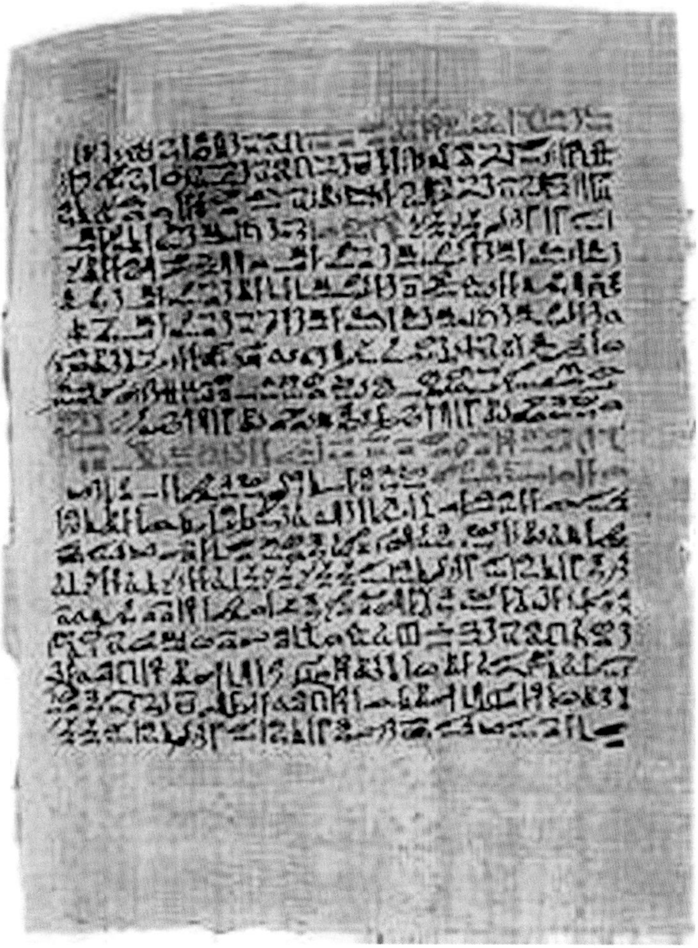

FIGURE 1.1 Ebers papyrus. Descriptions of chest pain associated with heart conditions and death can be found in ancient Egyptian writings. The Ebers papyrus is an Egyptian medical papyrus from c. 1550 BC. Among the oldest and most important medical papyri of ancient Egypt, it was acquired by Georg Ebers at Luxor (Thebes) in 1873–1874

that angina pectoris and angina tonsilaris were directly related [2]. Galen referred to angina as "cardalgia" based on the fact that the innervation of both heart and stomach were similar, and epigastric pain and tachycardia were considered to be the result of a "sympathetic" radiation from the heart or the stomach [3].

In the late eighteenth Century the work of British physicians triggered an evolution in the clinical understanding of angina pectoris, and its link with coronary artery disease. The term "angina pectoris" was first brought to the attention of the medical profession by William Heberden in 1768, when he presented his paper "Some Account of the Disorder of the Breast", to the Royal College of Physicians in London. Heberden's observations were based on an initial study of 20 cases. By the time he had incorporated the description in his book, "Commentaries on the History and Cure of Diseases", the number of cases had reached 100 [4]. Despite his excellent clinical description of angina pectoris, Heberden had not established a link between the symptom of "angina" and heart disease. As he admitted: "what the particular mischief is, is not easy to guess and I have had no opportunity of knowing with certainty;.... The pulse is sometimes not disturbed by this pain and consequently the heart is not affected by it" [4]. Edward Jenner (Fig. 1.2), at St George's Hospital in London, was responsible for the first suggestion that there was a probable association between coronary artery disease and angina pectoris. In 1776 he described autopsy findings compatible with coronary atheroma in two patients who had died from unknown causes: "a kind of fleshy tube formed within the vessels with a considerable quantity of ossific material dispersed irregularly through it." John Hunter (Fig. 1.3), a great surgeon and physician who suffered from angina, was the first to suggest the role of emotions in promoting an attack, and declared that his life was "in the hands of any rascal who chose to annoy and tease me". Rather amazingly, Hunter died suddenly following an argument with a colleague at

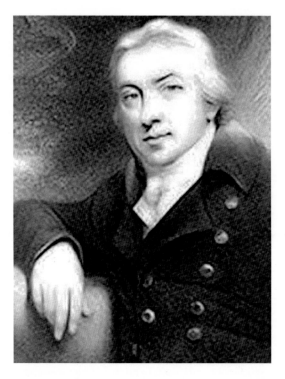

FIGURE 1.2 Jenner. Edward Jenner was born on 17 May 1749 in Berkeley, Gloucestershire, as the eighth of nine children. His father was the Reverend Stephen Jenner, the vicar of Berkeley. He obtained his MD from the University of St Andrew's in 1792. Jenner contributed to the understanding of angina pectoris but is renowned for his observation that milkmaids were generally immune to smallpox and for postulating that the pus in the blisters that milkmaids received from cowpox protected them from smallpox. In 1796, Jenner inoculated James Phipps, an 8-year-old boy, with pus scraped from cowpox blisters on the hands of Sarah Nelmes, a milkmaid who had caught cowpox from a cow called Blossom. The cow's hide can now be seen on the wall of the St George's Medical School library in Tooting, London. Jenner re-challenged Phipps and other subjects who were also inoculated to prove that they were immune to smallpox

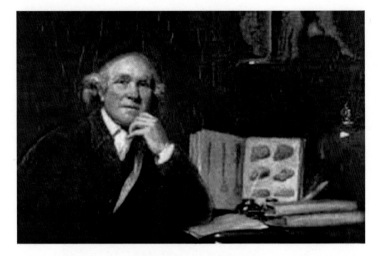

Figure 1.3 John Hunter. John Hunter (13 February 1728–16 October 1793) was one of the most distinguished scientists and surgeons of his time. He was a teacher and a friend of Edward Jenner. Hunter was elected Fellow of the Royal Society in 1767 and at this time he was considered the leading authority on venereal diseases. He however erroneously believed that gonorrhoea and syphilis were caused by the same agent. In 1768 Hunter was appointed as surgeon to St George's Hospital and in 1776 he was appointed surgeon to King George III. Hunter suffered from angina pectoris and his death in 1793 was apparently caused by a heart attack during an argument at St George's Hospital over the admission of students

St. George's Hospital in London, and coronary atheromatous disease was revealed on post-mortem examination. In 1809 a lecturer in anatomy in Glasgow, Allan Burns, suggested that myocardial ischaemia was the cause of angina pectoris. He indicated the importance of an adequate coronary blood supply for normal cardiac function, stating that "ossified coronary arteries" impaired the blood supply to the heart muscle [4]. Interestingly, the possibility that "spasm of the heart" could be the mechanism responsible for angina was initially put forward by Heberden, and Lauder Brunton considered the hypothesis that spasms of the coronary vessels were responsible for the condition. The vasomotor hypothesis was formalised by Knoknagal in 1867, who suggested that the symptoms of angina were caused by generalized arterial spasm. The link between coronary artery occlusions (thrombosis) and angina was confirmed at post mortem by Hannah in 1876, and in 1880 Vigerdt made the first full description of a myocardial infarction [4]. Albeit – over millennia – many 'remedies' were proposed for the management of angina. The first significant advance in the treatment of angina pectoris took place in 1867 when Brunton reported his observation that amyl nitrite was useful for the relief of angina symptoms. Later, in 1879 Morrell's paper in the *Lancet* described the beneficial effects of nitroglycerine in angina patients, as summarised by A. Leach [4].

Epidemiology: Age and Gender Differences

The prevalence and incidence of "stable angina pectoris" have been extremely difficult to establish over the years, as authors usually consider different definitions for the condition. Some use data representing subjects with chest pain and documented coronary artery disease, while others refer to typical chest discomfort and signs of myocardial ischaemia as entry criteria. Thus numbers vary considerably among reports depending on the definition of "angina" given. Importantly, the problem is further complicated by the fact that there has been a tendency to consider angina pain and obstructive coronary artery disease as synonymous. Statistical tools such as the Rose angina questionnaire have been helpful to standardise diagnostic criteria, to some degree. The problem, however, is that when sensitivity and specificity figures are established for these instruments the "gold standard" is the presence of "obstructive" coronary disease rather than myocardial ischaemia. Clinical tools, such as chest pain characteristics and the Rose questionnaire, have a reduced sensitivity and specificity compared with more objective diagnostic tests such as ECG findings, echocardiographic wall motion abnormalities, perfusion defects, or coronary arteriograpy [5]. The crucial issue is in establishing which "goldstandard" should be used; is it obstructive coronary artery disease or myocardial ischaemia that defines angina pectoris?

According to relatively recent publications [6–11], as summarised in the 2013 ESC guidelines for management of stable angina pectoris [12], the prevalence of angina increases with age in both men and women: from 5–7 % in women aged 45–64 years to 10–12 % in women aged 65–84 and from 4–7 % in men aged 45–64 years to 12–14 % in men aged 65–84 [6, 13]. It is conceivable that the improved sensitivity of contemporary diagnostic tools may contribute to the high prevalence of angina associated with coronary artery disease. The increased prevalence of the symptom of angina pectoris observed in middle-aged women compared with men, has been suggested to be due to a higher prevalence of the so called 'microvascular angina' in women [7, 8]. Unfortunately, little information is available at present regarding the prevalence of microvascular angina and coronary artery spasm in western populations. The annual incidence of stable angina pectoris in men aged 45–65 years, in western countries, has been estimated to be in the region of 1.0 % [6, 9]. The total incidence of angina, however, increases steeply with age in both men and women, reaching almost 4 % in people 75–84 years of age [9]. Of interest, epidemiological studies have shown that the incidence of angina pectoris parallels coronary artery disease mortality in multiple countries [9, 10]. A trend toward decreased coronary artery disease mortality (annual rates) has been reported recently by the American Heart Association [11]. Data in 2004 suggested that despite the declining incidence of myocardial infarction, the prevalence of angina remained high and direct costs in the USA in the year 2000 were estimated at up to $75 billion [14]. A more recent estimate of direct and indirect costs associated with the diagnosis and management stable angina in the USA [15] showed figures in the region of $177 billion.

The importance of stable angina from a public health perspective, particularly among women, is poorly understood and therefore continues to be debated. Coronary disease is the most common cause of women's death in developed countries [16], with stable angina as the most common clinical presentation within this demographic [17]. There is an apparent paradox, represented by the fact that angina prevalence in women is similar to that in men [18] despite the fact that men have an excess incidence of angiographically demonstrated coronary artery disease [19] and myocardial infarction [20].

A prospective cohort study by Hemingway et al. [9] used nationally linked registries in Finland, where the prevalence of angina in the general population is similar to that of the United States (5.4 % vs 6.3 % in women and 4.4 % vs 4.3 % in men, respectively) [21, 22], to contribute significantly to this debate. They assessed gender differences in chronic stable angina regarding incidence of angina in the general population, coronary mortality compared with the general population, and coronary event rates. Among patients aged 45–89 years who had no history of coronary disease, they defined new cases of "nitrate angina" based on nitrate prescription (56,441 women and 34,885 men) or "test-positive angina" based on abnormal invasive or noninvasive test results (11,391 women and 15,806 men). Patients were assessed between January 1, 1996, and December 31, 1998 and were follow-up until December 2001. Main outcome measures were coronary mortality at 4 years (n = 7906 deaths), and fatal or nonfatal myocardial infarction at 1 year (n = 3129 events). The main results of the study, as summarised by the authors, were as follows: age-standardized annual incidence (per 100 population of all cases of angina) was 2.03 in men and 1.89 in women, with a sex ratio of 1.07 (95 % confidence interval [CI], 1.06–1.09). At every age, "nitrate angina" in women and men was associated with a similar increase in risk of coronary mortality relative to the general population. Women with "test-positive angina" who were <75 years had higher coronary-standardized mortality ratios than men; for example, among those aged 55–64 years, it was 4.69 (95 % CI, 3.60–6.11) in women compared with 2.40 (95 % CI, 2.11–2.73) in men ($p<.001$ for interaction). There was a strong, graded relationship between amount of nitrates used and event rates; women using higher doses of nitrates had prognoses comparable with those of men. Among patients with diabetes and "test-positive angina", age-standardized coronary event rates were 9.9 per 100 person-years in women vs 9.3 in men ($p=.69$), and the fully adjusted male-female sex ratio was 1.07 (95% CI, 0.81–1.41). Based on these findings Hemingway et al. [9] concluded that: (1) women have a similarly high incidence of stable angina compared with men, (2) stable angina in women is associated with increased coronary mortality compared with women in the general population and, (3) among easily identifiable clinical subgroups, women have similarly high absolute rates of prognostic outcomes compared with men. Findings in this study [9] are important as Hemingway et al. have shown that, in the general population, angina in women occurs as commonly as in men, and its prognostic impact suggests that it should not be discounted as a benign or soft diagnosis. This study highlights the public health importance of angina in women and the importance of understanding the mechanisms underlying some of the gender discrepancies in incidence and outcome.

References

1. Deines, H, Grapow, H, Westendorf W. Grundriß der Medizin der alten Ägypter. IV. D. Magen-Herz. Berlin: Akademie Verlag; 1958. p. 88–100.
2. Heusch B, Guth BD, Heusch G. Pathophysiology and rational pharmacotherapy of myocardial ischemia. A brief history of angina pectoris: change of concepts and ideas. Springer-Verlag New York 1990
3. Siegel RE. (Galen),+GALEN, Siegel RE: Galen on surgery of the pericardium: an early record of therapy based on anatomic and experimental studies. Am J Cardiol. 1970;26:524–7.
4. Kaufman DMH, Ewart DRBL, Hunter RD, Leach MA, Fulton DWFM, Rees DJR, Arnott PM, Gorlin DR, Bent P, Muller O, Morris PJN, Oliver DMF, Michael SJ, Friesinger GC,

Borchgrevink CF, Julian DDG. Res Medica, April 1967, Special Issue – Lauder Brunton Centenary Symposium on Angina Pectoris. Res Medica. 1:1–70. http://dx.doi.org/10.2218/resmedica.v0i0.473

5. Rose GA, Blackburn H. Cardiovascular survey methods. Monogr Ser World Health Organ. 1968;56:1–188.
6. National Institutes of Health. Morbidity & mortality: 2012 chart book on cardiovascular, lung, and blood diseases. Bethesda: National Institutes of Health; 2012. p. 116.
7. Reis SE, Holubkov R, Conrad Smith AJ, Kelsey SF, Sharaf BL, Reichek N, Rogers WJ, Merz CN, Sopko G, Pepine CJ. Coronary microvascular dysfunction is highly prevalent in women with chest pain in the absence of coronary artery disease: results from the NHLBI WISE study. Am Heart J. 2001;141:735–41.
8. Han SH, Bae JH, Holmes DRJ, Lennon RJ, Eeckhout E, Barsness GW, Rihal CS, Lerman A. Sex differences in atheroma burden and endothelial function in patients with early coronary atherosclerosis. Eur Heart J. 2008;29:1359–69.
9. Hemingway H, McCallum A, Shipley M, Manderbacka K, Martikainen P, Keskimaki I. Incidence and prognostic implications of stable angina pectoris among women and men. JAMA. 2006;295:1404–11.
10. Ducimetiere P, Ruidavets JB, Montaye M, Haas B, Yarnell J. Five-year incidence of angina pectoris and other forms of coronary heart disease in healthy men aged 50-59 in France and Northern Ireland: the Prospective Epidemiological Study of Myocardial Infarction (PRIME) Study. Int J Epidemiol. 2001;30:1057–62.
11. Roger VL, Go AS, Lloyd-Jones DM, Benjamin EJ, Berry JD, Borden WB, Bravata DM, Dai S, Ford ES, Fox CS, Fullerton HJ, Gillespie C, Hailpern SM, Heit JA, Howard VJ, Kissela BM, Kittner SJ, Lackland DT, Lichtman JH, Lisabeth LD, Makuc DM, Marcus GM, Marelli A, Matchar DB, Moy CS, Mozaffarian D, Mussolino ME, Nichol G, Paynter NP, Soliman EZ, et al. Heart disease and stroke statistics – 2012 update: a report from the American Heart Association. Circulation. 2012;125:e2–e220.
12. Montalescot G, Sechtem U, Achenbach S, Andreotti F, Arden C, Budaj A, Bugiardini R, Crea F, Cuisset T, Di Mario C, Ferreira JR, Gersh BJ, Gitt AK, Hulot JS, Marx N, Opie LH, Pfisterer M, Prescott E, Ruschitzka F, Sabaté M, Senior R, Taggart DP, Van Der Wall EE, Vrints CJM, Zamorano JL, Baumgartner H, Bax JJ, Bueno H, Dean V, Deaton C, et al. 2013 ESC guidelines on the

management of stable coronary artery disease. Eur Heart J. 2013;34:2949–3003.

13. Zaher C, Goldberg GA, Kadlubek P. Estimating angina prevalence in a managed care population. Am J Manag Care. 2004;10:S339–46.

14. Javitz HS, Ward MM, Watson JB, Jaana M. Cost of illness of chronic angina. Am J Manag Care. 2004;10:S358–69.

15. Fihn SD, Gardin JM, Abrams J, Berra K, Blankenship JC, Dallas AP, Douglas PS, Foody JM, Gerber TC, Hinderliter AL, King SB, Kligfield PD, Krumholz HM, Kwong RYK, Lim MJ, Linderbaum JA, Mack MJ, Munger MA, Prager RL, Sabik JF, Shaw LJ, Sikkema JD, Smith CRJ, Smith SCJ, Spertus JA, Williams SV. ACCF/AHA/ACP/AATS/PCNA/SCAI/STS guideline for the diagnosis and management of patients with stable ischemic heart disease: a report of the American College of Cardiology Foundation/American Heart Association Task Force on Practice Guidelines, and the American College of Physicians, American Association for Thoracic Surgery, Preventive Cardiovascular Nurses Association, Society for Cardiovascular Angiography and Interventions, and Society of Thoracic Surgeons. J Am Coll Cardiol. 2012;60:e44–e164.

16. Casper ML, Barnett E, Halverson JA, et al. Women and heart disease: an atlas of racial and ethnic disparities in mortality. Morgantown: Office for Social Environment and Health Research, West Virginia University; 2000.

17. Murabito JM, Evans JC, Larson MG, Levy D. Prognosis after the onset of coronary heart disease. An investigation of differences in outcome between the sexes according to initial coronary disease presentation. Circulation. 1993;88:2548–55.

18. Reunanen A, Aromaa A, Pyorala K, Punsar S, Maatela J, Knekt P. The Social Insurance Institution's coronary heart disease study. Baseline data and 5-year mortality experience. Acta Med Scand Suppl. 1983;673:1–120.

19. Bugiardini R, Bairey Merz CN. Angina with 'normal' coronary arteries: a changing philosophy. JAMA. 2005;293:477–84.

20. Tunstall-Pedoe H, Kuulasmaa K, Mahonen M, Tolonen H, Ruokokoski E, Amouyel P. Contribution of trends in survival and coronary-event rates to changes in coronary heart disease mortality: 10-year results from 37 WHO MONICA project populations. Monitoring trends and determinants in cardiovascular disease. Lancet. 1999;353:1547–57.

21. Crea F. Chronic ischaemic heart disease. In: ESC textbook of cardiology. Oxford: Oxford University Press; 2010.
22. Hamm CW, Bassand J-P, Agewall S, Bax J, Boersma E, Bueno H, Caso P, Dudek D, Gielen S, Huber K, Ohman M, Petrie MC, Sonntag F, Uva MS, Storey RF, Wijns W, Zahger D. ESC Guidelines for the management of acute coronary syndromes in patients presenting without persistent ST-segment elevation: the Task Force for the management of acute coronary syndromes (ACS) in patients presenting without persistent ST-segment elevation. Eur Heart J. 2011;32:2999–3054.

Chapter 2
Stable Angina Pectoris: Definition, Clinical Presentation and Pathophysiologic Mechanisms

Abstract Angina is usually caused by coronary artery disease; atherosclerotic plaques in the coronary arteries cause progressive narrowing of the arterial lumen and symptoms occur when the restricted blood flow does not provide adequate amounts of oxygen to the myocardium during oxygen demand increases (such as during exercise). Angina can also, less commonly, be caused by: valve disease (for example aortic stenosis), hypertrophic obstructive cardiomyopathy, or hypertensive heart disease. This classical definition of angina pectoris is applicable, essentially and almost exclusively, to myocardial ischaemia caused by obstructive coronary atherosclerosis. Therefore, it does not necessarily encompass all of the various presentations of angina pectoris identified over the past five decades. Dynamic, functional mechanisms may play a key role in the genesis of angina both in the presence and the absence of epicardial coronary artery obstructions. This chapter will discuss the different forms of clinical presentation of angina pectoris and the various pathophysiological mechanisms responsible for the occurrence of myocardial ischaemia. In addition, the concept of coronary flow reserve, haemodynamic assessment of coronary artery stenosis and the role that abnormalities

J.C. Kaski, *Essentials in Stable Angina Pectoris*,
DOI 10.1007/978-3-319-41180-4_2,
© Springer International Publishing Switzerland 2016

in cardiac metabolism can play in exacerbating myocardial ischaemia will be also addressed in this chapter.

Definition, clinical presentation and pathophysiology

The UK National Institute for Clinical Excellence (NICE) defines angina pectoris as "chest pain (or constricting discomfort) caused by an insufficient blood supply to the heart muscle. Angina is usually caused by coronary artery disease; atherosclerotic plaques in the coronary arteries cause progressive narrowing of the lumen, and symptoms occur when the restricted blood flow does not provide adequate amounts of oxygen to the myocardium during oxygen demand increases (such as during exercise). Angina can also, less commonly, be caused by: valve disease (for example aortic stenosis), hypertrophic obstructive cardiomyopathy, or hypertensive heart disease" [1]. This classical definition of angina pectoris is applicable, essentially and almost exclusively, to myocardial ischaemia caused by obstructive coronary atherosclerosis. Therefore, it does not necessarily encompass all of the various presentations of angina pectoris identified over the past five decades. NICE's characterization of angina [1], similar to other angina guidelines on both sides of the Atlantic, pivots on the primacy of atherosclerotic plaque as the cause of myocardial ischaemia. In my view, this paradigm needs to be revised, as rapidly emerging evidence indicates that angina pectoris (hence myocardial ischaemia) can result from several mechanisms, not all of which necessarily involving obstructive coronary artery disease.

Stable angina usually occurs predictably, with physical exertion or emotional stress, and is relieved within minutes of rest. The characteristic chest pain (angina pectoris) of stable angina is triggered by an imbalance between myocardial oxygen demand and myocardial oxygen supply, which results in myocardial ischaemia. Anginal pain results from the release of metabolites (such as adenosine) during ischaemia, which stimulate sensitive nerve endings, sending appropriate signals to relevant centres in the brain [2]. Patients with stable angina pectoris typically present with effort induced angina that is often reproducible, i.e. occurring consistently at similar levels of exertion, and relieved by rest and sublingual nitrates (Box 2.1). This type of presentation is commonly seen in patients with obstructive coronary artery stenoses that limit the ability of the coronary circulation to meet an increased myocardial oxygen demand. It is not infrequent, however, for patients with stable angina to develop episodes of chest pain at rest or with variable degrees of effort, including minimal exertion. This indicates the presence of a variable "threshold" for angina without necessarily reflecting that the condition has become "unstable". Such a variable threshold for angina is the result of dynamic changes in the coronary circulation. For example, increases in vasomotor tone result in post stenotic pressure loss (i.e. turbulent flow): likewise, either focal or diffuse spasm can take place at the site of a coronary artery stenosis or in non-stenotic segments of a diseased epicardial artery [3]. Thus different pathophysiological mechanisms determine the different clinical presentations of stable angina seen in day-to-day clinical practice. These mechanisms will be discussed in subsequent chapters.

Box 2.1. Characteristics of typical angina according to the National Institute for Clinical Excellence (NICE), UK

Angina Pectoris is characterised by the following attributes:

1. **Constricting discomfort in the front of the chest, in the neck, shoulders, jaw, or arms.**
2. **Precipitated by physical exertion.**
3. **Relieved by rest or glyceryl trinitrate (GTN) within about 5 min.**

People with typical angina have all three of the above features.

People with atypical angina have two of the above features.

People with non-anginal chest pain have one or none of the above features.

Importantly, myocardial ischaemia can, and often does, occur in the absence of chest pain (silent myocardial ischaemia) due to the impaired transmission of painful stimuli to the cortex (and other unidentified mechanisms). Silent ischaemia should not be confused with coronary artery disease (coronary stenosis) that is not severe enough to cause myocardial ischaemia. Indeed, many patients have coronary artery disease, reducing the coronary lumen diameter by varying degrees (diagnosed by angiography), that does not affect coronary blood supply and hence does not trigger angina pectoris.

Characteristics of Stable Angina Pain: Typical and Atypical Angina Pectoris and Non-cardiac Chest Pain

Irrespective of the underlying pathogenic mechanisms, the chest pain (angina pectoris) resulting from myocardial ischaemia has typical characteristics that help physicians to identify the potentially ischaemic nature of the symptom. The chest discomfort associated with myocardial ischaemia is often analysed in relation to four characteristics, to establish whether it represents typical angina and, as such, suggests the possibility of myocardial ischaemia and/or coronary artery disease. The character, location and duration of the chest discomfort, as well as its relationship to exertion and relieving factors, are important to identify what constitute typical and atypical angina pectoris. Typically, angina is described not necessarily as "pain" but as a "discomfort"; a feeling of pressure, tightness or heaviness. Patients often use the words "strangling", "constricting," and "oppressive," to describe the symptom. The discomfort caused by myocardial ischaemia is usually located in the centre of the chest, over the sternum. However, patients commonly mention other locations such as the epigastrium, the throat, the lower jaw or teeth, the area between the shoulder blades or the arms, the wrists and, less commonly, the fingers. Shortness of breath can also frequently occur in association with angina.

More rarely, patients report fatigue, nausea, and a sense of impending doom during episodes of myocardial ischaemia. On occasion, shortness of breath may be the sole symptom reflecting ischaemia, and this poses a diagnostic problem. The duration of the chest discomfort is usually short, typically dissipating within 10 min. Importantly, chest pain lasting just a few seconds is unlikely to be caused by myocardial ischaemia. Angina is classically triggered by exercise, particularly by walking uphill, and/or by emotional stress. Angina commonly increases in severity with increasing levels of exertion, and many patients report worse chest discomfort when exercising in cold weather or after meals. Albeit typical effort related angina tends to recur with similar degrees of activity, a variable threshold for angina has been described, particularly in relation to coronary vasomotor mechanisms taking place at the site of a coronary stenosis [3]. An important diagnostic feature of typical angina is that the discomfort or pain is relieved rapidly after the cessation of the effort that triggered the symptom, and that buccal or sublingual nitrates rapidly relieve the anginal symptoms. The characteristics of typical and atypical angina, as suggested by Diamond [4] are summarized in Box 2.2. When all three criteria are present, the diagnosis of typical angina is made; but although typical angina is markedly suggestive of myocardial ischaemia, this does not necessarily mean that such symptoms can only be caused by obstructive atherosclerotic coronary artery disease. Typical angina can also be seen in patients with microvascular angina, in the absence of coronary atherosclerosis [5]. Atypical angina meets only two of the three criteria summarised in Box 2.1. Atypical angina generally resembles typical angina regarding location, character, and response to nitrates, but it is not necessarily triggered by effort. Often, atypical pain is described as developing at rest ("out the blue", as often referred to by patients), increasing in severity gradually and steadily, then slowly decreasing in intensity after 5–15 min. This type of anginal pain is common in patients with Prinzmetal's variant angina [6]. Prolonged pain, occurring during or after exertion, and showing a poor response to the administration of sublingual nitrates, is suggestive of microvascular angina [7].

Box 2.2. Diamond's suggested classification of chest pain for the diagnosis of angina pectoris (Ref. [4])

- **Typical (definite angina):**
  - **Substernal discomfort with characteristic quality and duration,**
  - **Provoked by exertion or emotional stress,**
  - **Relieved by rest or short-acting nitrate drug.**

The characteristic quality of the pain in stable angina is dull, heavy, or aching (not sharp or burning), and its duration should be minutes (not seconds or hours).
- **Atypical (probable angina) meets two of the above criteria.**
- **Non-cardiac chest pain meets one or none of the above criteria.**

These criteria aim at identifying angina pectoris triggered by obstructive coronary artery disease

---

Pathophysiology of Angina and Different Types of Stable Angina Pectoris

Myocardial ischemia is caused by an imbalance between myocardial oxygen supply and myocardial metabolic demand. Reduced coronary blood supply, excessive increase in myocardial oxygen demand, and/or a combination of these mechanisms, represent the most common pathogenesis of angina pectoris. In many instances, the development of exertional angina pectoris, or its exacerbation, is associated with the presence of severe anaemia, hyperthyroidism, or other systemic conditions that may affect the myocardial oxygen supply/demand balance.

Discussion of these secondary forms of angina is beyond the scope of this chapter, but will be mentioned briefly throughout the text.

Reduced Myocardial Oxygen Supply due to Coronary Artery Stenosis

The delivery of appropriate myocardial blood supply is dependent on the integrity of both the coronary conduit vessels i.e. the epicardial coronary arteries, and the coronary microvascular circulation. Obstructions to coronary blood flow by coronary atheromatous plaques affecting conduit coronary arteries is the most common cause of chronic stable angina. However, functional phenomena such as increased vasoconstriction affecting the epicardial arteries also contribute significantly [3]. Similarly, functional and organic abnormalities affecting the coronary microcirculation can lead to angina pectoris ('microvascular angina'), which can be indistinguishable from that caused by epicardial coronary artery disease [8, 9].

Obstructions to coronary blood flow can be 'fixed', such as those caused by epicardial atherosclerotic plaques encroaching upon the lumen of the vessel, or 'dynamic', as seen in patients with Prinzmetal's variant angina. In the latter, coronary artery spasm can interrupt epicardial coronary blood flow and lead to myocardial ischemia in the absence of increased myocardial oxygen demand [3]. In some patients with stable angina, fixed and dynamic obstructions may coexist, leading to the development of variable threshold exertional angina ('mixed angina') [10].

Fixed Coronary Obstructions Caused by Atheromatous Plaques

Atheromatous plaques limiting coronary blood flow in large epicardial coronary arteries are a very common cause of angina pectoris. Progressive atheroma formation leads to geometric changes in the vessel wall ('vascular remodeling') which is associated with inflammatory mechanisms and oxidative stress in addition to hemodynamic changes.

Remodeling can be either "positive", when the plaque grows towards the adventitia and the lumen size is maintained by a compensatory enlargement of the vessel wall area facilitated by the elastic external membrane, as proposed by Glagov et al. [11], or "negative," when the atheromatous plaque impinges upon the arterial lumen and reduces the diameter of the coronary vessel. When obstructive coronary stenoses offer substantial resistance to blood flow, the driving pressure drops distally to the stenosis. As driving pressure is a major determinant of blood flow, significant pressure drop distal to a stenosis can reduce blood supply and trigger myocardial ischaemia. Under baseline conditions, unless the obstructive plaque is extremely severe, pressure drops are compensated for by a parallel reduction of distal coronary resistance, via dilatation of arteriolar vessels. Experimental studies [12] have shown that coronary blood flow starts being affected when epicardial artery lumen diameter is reduced by >50 %. In dogs, a reduction of 85–90 % in coronary artery diameter is required to cause myocardial ischemia at rest (Fig. 2.1). Obviously, marked increases in myocardial oxygen demand can trigger ischaemia with lesser degrees of coronary obstruction.

--→

FIGURE 2.1 Relation between coronary flow and degree of stenosis in the intact coronary bed (Ref. [12]). Flow under resting conditions is designated by an arbitrary level of 1.0. Degree of stenosis in this case is expressed in terms of reduction in luminal cross-section area, assuming concentric geometry; 30, 50, 70 and 90 % diameter stenosis would correspond to area reductions of 50, 75, 90, and 99 %, respectively. The *upper curve* and data points represent maximal possible flow when coronary reserve is fully utilized, that is, flow during maximal vasodilation at a normal aortic pressure. The curve has been derived from a large scale model of the coronary circulation, instrumented to permit detailed pressure and velocity measurements before, within and beyond stenosis of different configuration (here concentric). The data points are derived from *in vivo* studies of artificial stenosis in dogs by Gould and Furuse and their co-workers. The *lower line* and data points are control values from the same studies, that is, values before vasodilation with normal autoregulatroy mechanisms intact

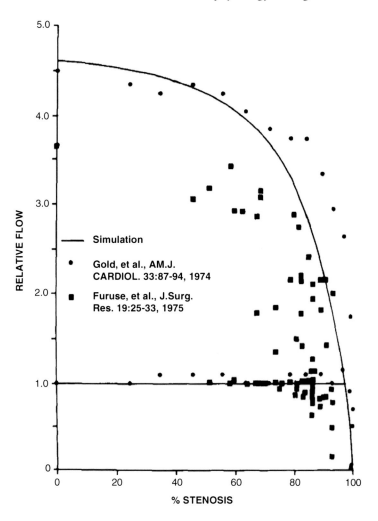

How to Assess the Haemodynamic Effect of a Coronary Stenosis

The hemodynamic relevance of a coronary stenosis can now be accurately assessed during coronary angiography, using quantitative measurement of *fractional flow reserve* (FFR) [13]. FFR is calculated as the ratio between the mean pressures distal and proximal to the stenosis during maximal vasodilatation (usually induced by intracoronary administration of adenosine). An FFR <0.80 is considered to identify flow-limiting stenosis able to cause myocardial ischemia during increased myocardial oxygen consumption. Although FFR can be affected by collateral circulation, baseline microvascular constriction, preload, and after load, it represents a major improvement as compared with the more subjective visual evaluation of stenosis severity. However, clinical trials have failed to demonstrate that FFR guided revascularisation results in improved clinical outcomes [14]. In the clinical setting, the presence, degree, and extent of coronary stenoses, and their impact on myocardial ischemia in the relevant myocardial territory, is useful to characterise the haemodynamic impact of a given coronary stenosis.

Coronary flow reserve (CFR) can also be used to assess the hemodynamic significance of a stenosis. CFR is expressed as the ratio between coronary blood flow velocity during maximal coronary vasodilatation (induced by adenosine) and flow velocity at baseline, as assessed by intracoronary Doppler recording. A CFR >2.5 as measured by this method, is consider to be normal [15].

The Role of Collateral Circulation

Collateral vessels can be present in patients with obstructive coronary artery disease. These vessels develop mainly from pre-existing inter-coronary arterial conduits, which further develop as a result of the pressure gradient that exists between the normal vessel from which they emerge, and the stenotic vessel they supply [16].

These preexisting conduits progressively develop into mature vessels, reaching diameters of up to 200–250 μm, with marked differences between the types and sizes of collateral vessels seen in different patients on angiography [17]. The collateral circulation may improve the ischaemic threshold and may also have a protective effect against ischaemia, manifest by reduced ischemia and infarct size following an acute coronary occlusion, as well as better LV function after myocardial revascularisation [18].

Dynamic Coronary Obstructions in the Epicardial Artery and the Microcirculation

Patients with Prinzmetal's variant angina (coronary artery spasm, the typical 'dynamic' coronary obstruction that can lead to myocardial ischemia and angina at rest) usually present with chest pain at rest associated with transient ST-segment elevation. Typical coronary spasm can be focal, affecting one or more segments in the epicardial arteries, or diffuse, affecting long segments of the vessel [6]. Patients experiencing these vessel spasms usually have a preserved exercise capacity; it is therefore unusual for this condition to manifest itself as chronic stable angina. Hence Prinzmetal's variant angina will not be discussed in detail in this book. Lesser degrees of coronary vasoconstriction can, however, occur at the site of eccentric atheromatous plaques in patients with exercise-induced stable angina, thus dynamically magnifying the coronary diameter reduction caused by the atheromatous coronary artery stenosis itself [3]. The coexistence of obstructive stenoses and dynamic vasomotor changes is not uncommon in patients with stable angina pectoris and is usually responsible for the variable angina threshold observed in many effort-induced stable angina patients [3, 10].

Increased Myocardial Oxygen Demand: The Role of Increased Heart Rate as a Trigger of Ischaemia and a Marker of Clinical Outcome

In daily life, myocardial oxygen demand increases in response to increased heart rate and/or increased left ventricular contractility. Similarly, any factors increasing left ventricular preload (e.g., increased end diastolic pressure or LV volume) or afterload (e.g., increased systolic blood pressure, arterial stiffness) will also cause an increase in myocardial oxygen demand [19]. Increases in myocardial oxygen demand, such as those associated with tachycardia, can trigger ischaemia in the presence of severe obstructive coronary artery disease. Heart rate is a major determinant of myocardial oxygen consumption, and elevated heart rate increases energy requirements and myocardial oxygen demand. Elevated heart rate shortens the length of each cardiac cycle, thereby reducing diastolic perfusion time and oxygen supply. Increased heart rate has been suggested to be a predictor of impaired clinical outcome [20–22].

A raised heart rate has also been suggested to increase endothelial shear stress, which may increase the risk of acute myocardial infarction by mechanically stressing atherosclerotic plaques [23, 24].

Heart rate increases thus appear to play an important role in the development and progression of coronary atherosclerosis as well as in triggering angina: via an increase in myocardial oxygen demand, a reduction in diastolic perfusion and increased shear stress.

Combined Pathogenic Mechanisms

Several clinical conditions can cause myocardial ischemia by affecting myocardial oxygen delivery and/or demand. Examples of these include: aortic valve stenosis, hypertension and hypertrophic cardiomyopathy (HCM). In HCM several mechanisms coexist that can lead to angina, such as left ventricular hypertrophy, microvascular remodeling, microvessel wall thickening, perivascular fibrosis, extravascular compression of the coronary microvasculature, etc. Conditions that increase myocardial metabolic demand, such as thyrotoxicosis, can also cause myocardial ischemia, particularly in the presence of coronary blood flow limiting stenoses. Clinical conditions such as amyloidosis, myxoedema and myocardial granuloma can affect microvascular function and oxygen delivery to the myocyte [25].

Metabolic and Functional Consequences of Transient Myocardial Ischemia

Ischemic episodes in patients with stable angina are usually transient and do not cause myocyte injury. More prolonged myocardial ischemia, however, can lead to alterations in cardiac metabolism, increased high sensitivity cardiac troponin levels, and left ventricular contractile abnormalities [19]. The transient cell swelling that accompanies myocardial ischemia causes ionic shifts and further ischaemia [19].

Impaired mitochondrial oxidative phosphorylation results in reduced levels of adenosine triphosphate (ATP), leading to acidosis and anaerobic metabolism.

The healthy heart derives most of its energy from the free fatty acid (FFA) pathway that accounts for approximately two-thirds of adenosine triphosphate (ATP) production. Glucose oxidation is another mechanism for myocardial energy production. During mild to moderate myocardial ischemia, the myocytes accelerate glucose uptake to generate sufficient ATP to maintain calcium homeostasis. During severe ischemia the myocardium gets most of its energy from beta-oxidation, which is associated with lactate production. Under these circumstances, FFA oxidation inhibits glucose oxidation via competitive interaction (Randle phenomenon). FFA oxidation generates more ATP compared with glucose oxidation, but more oxygen is consumed in the process and more reactive oxygen species (ROS) are generated with deleterious effects on mitochondrial efficiency [26–28].

The anaerobic state leads to increased fatty acid oxidation and intracellular acidosis, thus to an increase in intracellular sodium concentration [29]. Cellular sodium concentration increases in response to an exacerbated late sodium current activity (INaL) and influx of sodium ions via sodium – hydrogen exchange (NHE) pH dependent mechanisms [30, 31].

The increase in intracellular sodium results in Ca2+ overload, which impairs left ventricular relaxation, subsequently causing microvascular compression and ultimately leading to left ventricular dysfunction [32]. The cardiac ATP-sensitive potassium (KATP) channel is thought to have a cardioprotective role in ischemic conditions [33]. This channel shortens the cardiac action potential duration during ischemia and reduces the harmful Ca2+ influx [34]. These metabolic effects represent potential targets for drug therapy.

Coronary Microvascular Dysfunction Leading to Microvascular Angina

Abnormalities in the vasodilatory ability of the coronary microvasculature, generally due to endothelial dysfunction, can lead to myocardial ischemia (microvascular angina) even in the absence of epicardial coronary artery stenosis [5, 7–9]. Microvascular angina can develop in patients with cardiovascular risk factors such as hypertension, increased LDL cholesterol, obesity, diabetes and smoking. These risk factors increase oxidative stress within endothelial cells and impair both the bioavailability of nitric oxide (NO), a potent vasodilator agent produced by the endothelium, and the actions of endothelial nitric oxide synthase (eNOS), the enzyme responsible for the catalytic conversion of the amino acid substrate L-arginine into NO [35]. Endothelial dysfunction contributes significantly to the development of functional vasomotor abnormalities at both the epicardial and the microvascular levels.

The clinical significance of coronary microvascular dysfunction (CMD) has not been given as much attention as that of epicardial coronary artery stenoses/disease [5]. In recent years, however, it has become apparent that a condition often referred to as "angina with normal coronary arteries", "cardiac syndrome X" or "microvascular angina" is more common than initially thought, and is associated with impaired clinical outcomes in a sizeable proportion of patients. Coronary resistance is primarily controlled by the pre-arterioles (<500 μm in diameter) and arterioles (<200 μm). The arterioles are true intramyocardial vessels and represent the regulatory component of the coronary circulation, controlling over 55 % of the total coronary vascular resistance. Arterioles are subdivided, according to their diameter and the mechanisms that affect their tone, into larger, medium sized and smaller arterioles [9, 36] (Fig. 2.2).

Endothelium-dependent vasoreactivity prevails in the larger arterioles (100–200 μm in diameter). Medium-sized microvessels (40–100 μm in diameter) react predominantly to intraluminal pressure changes sensed by stretch receptors located in vascular smooth muscle cells (myogenic control). They constrict when the intraluminal pressure increases and, conversely, dilate when the pressure decreases [37]. Finally, the tone of the smaller arterioles (vessels <40 μm in diameter) is modulated by the metabolic activity of the myocardium. As such, increased metabolic activity leads to vasodilatation of the smaller arterioles, which leads to pressure reduction in the medium-sized microvessels and myogenic dilation. This, in turn, increases flow upstream, resulting in endothelium-dependent vasodilation [5]. These mechanisms allow the microcirculation to regulate myocardial perfusion both at rest and at different degrees of myocardial metabolic demand.

Structural and functional mechanisms altering the physiological function of the coronary microvasculature lead to CMD and angina pectoris. There are two main functional mechanisms responsible for microvascular angina: abnormal coronary vasodilation and microvascular coronary spasm [5, 9]. As recently reviewed by Crea et al. [38], evidence gathered

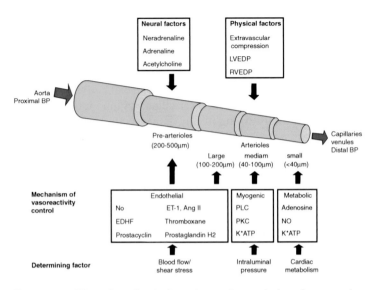

FIGURE 2.2 The microcirculation plays a key role in microvascular angina. Coronary blood flow is driven by the pressure difference between the aorta and the capillary bed and modulated further by various physical and neural factors, which affect the microcirculation. Moreover, the different compartments of the microcirculation are influenced by one main physiological mechanism to control their vascular tone with cardiac metabolism as the final determining factor (From Ref. [5] with permission)

over the past few years indicates that endothelium-independent microvascular dysfunction may also lead to abnormal CFR, as a result of functional and structural abnormalities that develop with aging and in the presence of hypertension, diabetes, dyslipidaemia, and insulin resistance. In fact, conditions such as hyperglycaemia, insulin resistance, and hyperinsulinaemia, can alter both endothelial-dependent and endothelial-independent coronary vasodilation. Therefore, interventions that improve insulin sensitivity can improve both endothelial dysfunction and myocardial ischaemia in patients experiencing angina in the absence of obstructive coronary atheromatous disease [38]. Moreover, chronic inflammation, as recently reviewed by Faccini et al. [39], is another important risk factor/mechanism of CMD. High C-reactive protein is correlated with an increased frequency of ischaemic episodes, as assessed by ambulatory ECG monitoring in patients with microvascular angina [40]. This suggests a role for inflammation in the modulation of the coronary microvascular circulation of such patients. Furthermore, and attesting to the pathogenic role of inflammation, CMD has recently been described both in patients with systemic lupus erythematosus and rheumatoid arthritis [41, 42].

Chronic Stable Angina Pectoris: Forms of Clinical Presentation

As a result of the pathophysiological mechanisms described above, two major forms of chronic stable angina pectoris can be identified – after excluding epicardial coronary artery spasm: Stable angina due to obstructive epicardial coronary artery disease and microvascular angina.

Diagnostic strategies, prognosis, and treatment of these two clinical presentations of stable angina will be discussed in subsequent chapters.

References

1. Cooper A, Calvert N, Skinner J, Sawyer L, Sparrow, K, Timmis A, Turnbull N, Cotterell M, Hill D, Adams P, Ashcroft J, Clark L, Coulden R, Hemingway H, James C, Jarman H, Kendall J, Lewis P, Patel K, Smeeth L, Taylor J. (2010). Chest pain of recent onset: Assessment and diagnosis of recent onset chest pain or discomfort of suspected cardiac origin London: National Clinical Guideli ne Centre for Acute and Chronic Conditions.
2. Crea F, Pupita G, Galassi AR, El-Tamimi H, Kaski JC, Davies G, Maseri A. Role of adenosine in pathogenesis of anginal pain. Circulation. 1990;81:164–72.

3. Maseri A, Davies G, Hackett D, Kaski JC. Coronary artery spasm and vasoconstriction. The case for a distinction. Circulation. 1990;81:1983–91.
4. Diamond GA. A clinically relevant classification of chest discomfort. J Am Coll Cardiol. 1983;1:574–5.
5. Herrmann J, Kaski JC, Lerman A. Coronary microvascular dysfunction in the clinical setting: from mystery to reality. Eur Heart J. 2012;33:2771–83.
6. Lanza GA, Sestito A, Sgueglia GA, Infusino F, Manolfi M, Crea F, Maseri A. Current clinical features, diagnostic assessment and prognostic determinants of patients with variant angina. Int J Cardiol. 2007;118:41–7.
7. Lanza GA, Crea F. Primary coronary microvascular dysfunction: clinical presentation, pathophysiology, and management. Circulation. 2010;121:2317–25.
8. Kaski JC. Pathophysiology and management of patients with chest pain and normal coronary arteriograms (cardiac syndrome X). Circulation. 2004;109:568–72.
9. Camici PG, Crea F. Coronary microvascular dysfunction. N Engl J Med. 2007;356:830–40.
10. Maseri A, Chierchia S, Kaski JC. Mixed angina pectoris. Am J Cardiol. 1985;56:30E–3.
11. Glagov S, Weisenberg E, Zarins CK, Stankunavicius R, Kolettis GJ. Compensatory enlargement of human atherosclerotic coronary arteries. N Engl J Med. 1987;316:1371–5.
12. Klocke FJ. Measurements of coronary blood flow and degree of stenosis: current clinical implications and continuing uncertainties. J Am Coll Cardiol. 1983;1:31–41.
13. De Bruyne B, Baudhuin T, Melin JA, Pijls NH, Sys SU, Bol A, Paulus WJ, Heyndrickx GR, Wijns W. Coronary flow reserve calculated from pressure measurements in humans. Validation with positron emission tomography. Circulation. 1994;89:1013–22.
14. De Bruyne B, Pijls NHJ, Kalesan B, Barbato E, Tonino PAL, Piroth Z, Jagic N, Mobius-Winkler S, Rioufol G, Witt N, Kala P, MacCarthy P, Engstrom T, Oldroyd KG, Mavromatis K, Manoharan G, Verlee P, Frobert O, Curzen N, Johnson JB, Juni P, Fearon WF. Fractional flow reserve-guided PCI versus medical therapy in stable coronary disease. N Engl J Med. 2012;367:991–1001.
15. Bach RG, Kern MJ. Practical coronary physiology. Clinical application of the Doppler flow velocity guide wire. Cardiol Clin. 1997;15:77–99.

16. Chilian WM, Mass HJ, Williams SE, Layne SM, Smith EE, Scheel KW. Microvascular occlusions promote coronary collateral growth. Am J Physiol. 1990;258:H1103–11.

17. Teunissen PFA, Horrevoets AJG, van Royen N. The coronary collateral circulation: genetic and environmental determinants in experimental models and humans. J Mol Cell Cardiol. 2012;52:897–904.

18. Kozman H, Cook JR, Wiseman AH, Dann RH, Engelman RM. Presence of angiographic coronary collaterals predicts myocardial recovery after coronary bypass surgery in patients with severe left ventricular dysfunction. Circulation. 1998;98:II57–61.

19. Pepine CJ, Nichols WW. The pathophysiology of chronic ischemic heart disease. Clin Cardiol. 2007;30:I4–9.

20. Diaz A, Bourassa MG, Guertin M-C, Tardif J-C. Long-term prognostic value of resting heart rate in patients with suspected or proven coronary artery disease. Eur Heart J. 2005;26:967–74.

21. Kolloch R, Legler UF, Champion A, Cooper-Dehoff RM, Handberg E, Zhou Q, Pepine CJ. Impact of resting heart rate on outcomes in hypertensive patients with coronary artery disease: findings from the INternational VErapamil-SR/trandolapril STudy (INVEST). Eur Heart J. 2008;29:1327–34.

22. Fox K, Borer JS, Camm AJ, Danchin N, Ferrari R, Lopez Sendon JL, Steg PG, Tardif J-C, Tavazzi L, Tendera M. Resting heart rate in cardiovascular disease. J Am Coll Cardiol. 2007;50:823–30.

23. Giannoglou GD, Chatzizisis YS, Zamboulis C, Parcharidis GE, Mikhailidis DP, Louridas GE. Elevated heart rate and atherosclerosis: an overview of the pathogenetic mechanisms. Int J Cardiol. 2008;126:302–12.

24. Heidland UE, Strauer BE. Left ventricular muscle mass and elevated heart rate are associated with coronary plaque disruption. Circulation. 2001;104:1477–82.

25. Naghavi M, Libby P, Falk E, Casscells SW, Litovsky S, Rumberger J, Badimon JJ, Stefanadis C, Moreno P, Pasterkamp G, Fayad Z, Stone PH, Waxman S, Raggi P, Madjid M, Zarrabi A, Burke A, Yuan C, Fitzgerald PJ, Siscovick DS, de Korte CL, Aikawa M, Airaksinen KEJ, Assmann G, Becker CR, Chesebro JH, Farb A, Galis ZS, Jackson C, Jang I-K, et al. From vulnerable plaque to vulnerable patient: a call for new definitions and risk assessment strategies: part II. Circulation. 2003;108:1772–8.

26. Stanley WC, Lopaschuk GD, Hall JL, McCormack JG. Regulation of myocardial carbohydrate metabolism under normal and isch-

aemic conditions. Potential for pharmacological interventions. Cardiovasc Res. 1997;33:243–57.

27. Stanley WC, Recchia FA, Lopaschuk GD. Myocardial substrate metabolism in the normal and failing heart. Physiol Rev. 2005;85:1093–129.

28. Jaswal JS, Keung W, Wang W, Ussher JR, Lopaschuk GD. Targeting fatty acid and carbohydrate oxidation – a novel therapeutic intervention in the ischemic and failing heart. Biochim Biophys Acta. 2011;1813:1333–50.

29. Hale SL, Shryock JC, Belardinelli L, Sweeney M, Kloner RA. Late sodium current inhibition as a new cardioprotective approach. J Mol Cell Cardiol. 2008;44:954–67.

30. Bers DM, Barry WH, Despa S. Intracellular Na+ regulation in cardiac myocytes. Cardiovasc Res. 2003;57:897–912.

31. Eigel BN, Hadley RW. Contribution of the Na(+) channel and Na(+)/H(+) exchanger to the anoxic rise of [Na(+)] in ventricular myocytes. Am J Physiol. 1999;277:H1817–22.

32. Silverman HS, Stern MD. Ionic basis of ischaemic cardiac injury: insights from cellular studies. Cardiovasc Res. 1994;28:581–97.

33. Kane GC, Liu X-K, Yamada S, Olson TM, Terzic A. Cardiac KATP channels in health and disease. J Mol Cell Cardiol. 2005;38:937–43.

34. Hibino H, Inanobe A, Furutani K, Murakami S, Findlay I, Kurachi Y. Inwardly rectifying potassium channels: their structure, function, and physiological roles. Physiol Rev. 2010;90:291–366.

35. Endemann DH, Schiffrin EL. Endothelial dysfunction. J Am Soc Nephrol. 2004;15:1983–92.

36. Patel B, Fisher M. Therapeutic advances in myocardial microvascular resistance: unravelling the enigma. Pharmacol Ther. 2010;127:131–47.

37. Kuo L, Chilian WM, Davis MJ. Coronary arteriolar myogenic response is independent of endothelium. Circ Res. 1990;66:860–6.

38. Crea F, Camici PG, Bairey Merz CN. Coronary microvascular dysfunction: an update. Eur Heart J. 2014;35:1101–11.

39. Faccini A, Kaski JC, Camici PG. Coronary microvascular dysfunction in chronic inflammatory rheumatoid diseases. Eur Heart J. 2016;37:1799–806. doi: 10.1093/eurheartj/ehw018.

40. Cosin-Sales J, Pizzi C, Brown S, Kaski JC. C-reactive protein, clinical presentation, and ischemic activity in patients with chest

pain and normal coronary angiograms. J Am Coll Cardiol. 2003;41:1468–74.

41. Ishimori ML, Martin R, Berman DS, Goykhman P, Shaw LJ, Shufelt C, Slomka PJ, Thomson LEJ, Schapira J, Yang Y, Wallace DJ, Weisman MH, Bairey Merz CN. Myocardial ischemia in the absence of obstructive coronary artery disease in systemic lupus erythematosus. JACC Cardiovasc Imaging. 2011;4:27–33.

42. Recio-Mayoral A, Rimoldi OE, Camici PG, Kaski JC. Inflammation and microvascular dysfunction in cardiac syndrome X patients without conventional risk factors for coronary artery disease. JACC Cardiovasc Imaging. 2013;6:660–7.

Chapter 3
Angina due to Obstructive Atherosclerotic Coronary Artery Disease: Diagnosis and Patient Risk Stratification

Abstract Chronic stable angina pectoris is the initial manifestation of ischemic heart disease in approximately 50 % of individuals. Exercise related angina caused by obstructive atherosclerotic coronary artery disease is the most common manifestation of ischaemic heart disease in men over 50 years of age and in post-menopausal women. Severe coronary artery stenoses resulting from atheromatous plaque growth can impair coronary blood flow supply to the myocardium, particularly when there is an increased myocardial oxygen demand. Patients who present with chest pain of suspected cardiac origin require accurate and timely diagnosis to guide the implementation of appropriate investigations and therapeutic interventions. Patient risk stratification is important in relation to strategic therapeutic decisions as well as the implementation of primary and secondary prevention. The importance of the clinical history as well as the appropriate use of diagnostic tests is the topic of this chapter.

Introduction

Effort induced angina caused by obstructive atherosclerotic coronary artery disease is the most common manifestation of ischaemic heart disease in men over 50 years of age and in

J.C. Kaski, *Essentials in Stable Angina Pectoris*,
DOI 10.1007/978-3-319-41180-4_3,
© Springer International Publishing Switzerland 2016

post-menopausal women. Chronic stable angina is the initial manifestation of ischemic heart disease in approximately one half of patients [1].

The pathogenesis of ischaemic heart disease involves inflammatory mechanisms, as well as endothelial activation and dysfunction (often linked to dyslipidaemia), which lead to the formation of atherosclerotic plaques in the coronary vessels and favour plaque growth, with subsequent disruption or erosion resulting in acute coronary events. A discussion of the molecular basis of atherosclerosis and cellular mechanisms of atherogenesis is beyond the remit of this book. The topic has been extensively reviewed in the literature over the past two decades [2–4].

Suffice it to say, however, that conventional risk factors play a major role in the development of coronary artery disease. Hypertension, hypercholesterolaemia, diabetes, sedentary lifestyle, obesity, smoking, and a family history of coronary disease all predispose to coronary epicardial and microvascular dysfunction, atheromatous plaque formation, and the progression of atherosclerosis [5–13].

Severe coronary stenoses resulting from atheromatous plaque growth can impair coronary blood flow supply to the myocardium, particularly when there is an increased myocardial oxygen demand (as discussed in Chap. 2). Establishing an accurate diagnosis of angina pectoris due to atheromatous coronary disease is a common challenge for all physicians, particularly cardiologists. This chapter focuses on the diagnosis of stable angina, the potentially serious complications of the condition and clinical outcomes in individuals affected by stable angina caused by atherosclerotic coronary artery disease. The content of this chapter is based mainly on current recommendations by the European Society of Cardiology [14].

Diagnosis

Patients who present with chest pain of suspected cardiac origin require accurate and timely diagnosis to guide the implementation of appropriate investigations and therapeutic interventions.

Current U.S. [1] and European [14] guidelines describe a range of potential noninvasive imaging and invasive modalities to assess patients with suspected stable angina pectoris due to coronary heart disease. In assessing patients presenting with angina pectoris, it is important to: (1) **establish an accurate diagnosis of myocardial ischaemia**; (2) **assess whether coronary artery disease is present and whether coronary artery stenoses are truly responsible for the patient's symptoms** and (3) **to risk stratify these individuals thoroughly**. All of these have importance for management and prognosis. Figure 3.1 shows the initial diagnostic algorithm proposed by the current guidelines of the ESC on management of stable angina pectoris.

Clinical History

A detailed clinical history remains one of the pillars of the diagnosis of angina pectoris. Although in a large proportion of cases it is possible to make a confident diagnosis of angina (caused by myocardial ischaemia) on the basis of the clinical history, including the characteristics of the chest discomfort, risk factors, past medical history and physical examination, confirming the diagnosis with objective tests and establishing the pathogenic mechanisms is necessary in most cases. The characteristics of typical and atypical angina have been described in Chap. 2. Physical examination can provide clues as to the presence of hyperlipidaemia, aortic valve disease, anaemia, heart failure, hypertension, peripheral vascular disease, and other conditions associated with angina and ischaemic heart disease.

The use of simple validated scores during the clinical consultation (considering age, gender, history of vascular disease, characteristics of the pain, and presence or absence of risk factors), allows an accurate ruling-out of coronary disease with a specificity of 81 % and a sensitivity of 87 % [15].

In patients with coronary artery disease, the severity of the ischaemic response can be characterised clinically using the classification proposed by the Canadian Cardiovascular Society. This classification, which for many years now has

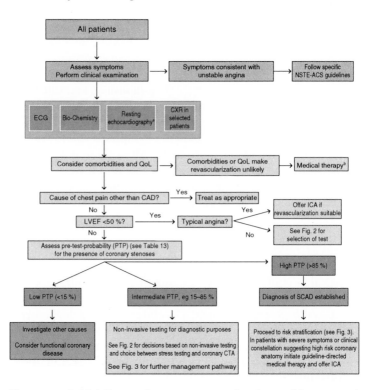

FIGURE 3.1 Initial diagnostic management of patients with suspected SCAD as suggested by the ESC guidelines (From Ref. [14], with permission). *CAD* coronary artery disease, *CTA* computed tomography angiography, *CXR* chest X-ray, *ECG* electrocardiogram, *ICA* invasive coronary angiography; *LVEF* left ventricular ejection fraction, *PTP* pre-test probability, *SCAD* stable coronary artery disease. ᵃMay be omitted in very young and healthy patients with a high suspicion of an extracardiac cause of chest pain and in multimorbid patients in which the echo result has no consequence for further patient management. ᵇIf diagnosis of SCAD is doubtful, establishing a diagnosis using pharmacologic stress imaging prior to treatment may be reasonable

been used worldwide as a grading system to establish the functional severity of stable angina [16], quantifies the threshold at which symptoms occur in relation to different degrees of physical activity (Box 3.1). It is, however, important to remember that many factors – not only coronary disease severity – can affect the angina class; therefore this classification is just an approximation as to the disease severity. Even in the absence of disease progression, functional class can vary significantly within individual patients due to the effect of dynamic factors.

Box 3.1. Canadian Cardiovascular Society Grading System for Stable Angina (Ref. [16])

Grade I

Grade I stable angina develops upon strenuous, rapid, and/or prolonged exertion during work or recreation but is not induced by ordinary physical activity, such as walking and climbing stairs.

Grade II

Grade II stable angina is characterized by a slight limitation of ordinary activity and is induced by the following:

- Walking or climbing stairs rapidly
- Walking uphill
- Walking or stair-climbing after meals
- Walking more than two level blocks or climbing more than one flight of ordinary stairs at a normal pace and in normal conditions
- Emotional stress
- During the few hours after waking

Grade III

Grade III stable angina is characterized by marked limitation of ordinary physical activity. It is induced by walking one or two level blocks and climbing one flight of stairs in normal conditions and at a normal pace.

Grade IV

Grade IV stable angina is characterized by an inability to carry on any physical activity without discomfort. Anginal syndrome may be present at rest.

Initial Basic Clinical Investigations

Baseline Electrocardiogram

A 12-lead ECG should be performed in all patients with chest pain suggestive of coronary artery disease, for patient characterisation (ESC recommendation class I C). More often than not, the baseline ECG will be normal if the patient is not experiencing any cardiac symptoms at the time of the test; occasionally, however, the baseline ECG may provide important diagnostic information. Importantly, a baseline 12-lead ECG may help to reach a diagnosis on the spot, if taken while the patient is experiencing his or her usual chest pain (i.e. ST-segment changes clearly showing myocardial ischaemia or diagnostic transient ST segment elevation in patients with coronary artery spasm – Prinzmetal's variant angina). The baseline ECG may also show other abnormalities that can guide the physician to the cause of the chest pain, such as: left ventricular hypertrophy, left or right bundle branch block (LBBB or RBBB), pre-excitation, atrial and ventricular arrhythmias, or conduction defects [14].

Blood Tests

Figure 3.2 illustrates the ESC recommendation level for different routine blood tests that can be carried out for assessment of stable angina, according to the ESC guidelines for the management of angina pectoris. Haemoglobin, plasma glucose, HbA1c, thyroid function (TSH), fasting lipid profile, tests of renal function, and liver function tests are all useful and easily obtainable basic screening tests that can help to identify secondary causes of (and triggers for) angina pectoris.

Baseline Echocardiogram and Cardiac Magnetic Resonance Imaging (CMRI)

Resting transthoracic echocardiography and CMRI provide information on cardiac structure and function. Regional wall

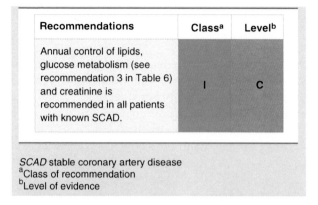

Recommendations	Class[a]	Level[b]
Annual control of lipids, glucose metabolism (see recommendation 3 in Table 6) and creatinine is recommended in all patients with known SCAD.	I	C

SCAD stable coronary artery disease
[a]Class of recommendation
[b]Level of evidence

FIGURE 3.2 Blood tests for routine re-assessment in patients with chronic stable coronary artery disease as recommended by the ESC guidelines on management of angina (From Ref. [14] with permission)

motion abnormalities detected on baseline echocardiographic assessment may alert one to the possibility of ischaemic heart disease. Other disorders that can be responsible for angina, such as aortic stenosis or hypertrophic cardiomyopathy, can be assessed objectively with an echocardiogram. Ventricular function, an important prognostic variable in patients with stable angina, can also be assessed thoroughly with the use of CMRI and echocardiography.

Continuous Ambulatory ECG Monitoring

Ambulatory ECG monitoring may show evidence of myocardial ischaemia during normal daily activities but it rarely adds important diagnostic information for stable angina patients, over and above that provided by the ECG stress test. However, it may reveal the occurrence of silent myocardial ischaemia [17] that can require further attention in a given patient. Ambulatory monitoring may be very useful in patients with arrhythmias and/or vasospastic angina pectoris, in whom episodes may occur unpredictably during any time of the day, and mainly at rest.

Diagnostic Tests for Myocardial Ischaemia and/or Coronary Artery Disease

For the use of diagnostic tests, the ESC recommends a Bayesian approach to the diagnosis of angina. This approach uses clinicians' pre-test estimates, i.e. pre-test probability (PTP) of disease, along with the results of diagnostic tests to generate individualized post-test disease probabilities for a given patient (Fig. 3.3). The PTP is influ-

	Typical angina		Atypical angina		Non-anginal pain	
Age	Men	Women	Men	Women	Men	Women
30–39	59	28	29	10	18	5
40–49	69	37	38	14	25	8
50–59	77	47	49	20	34	12
60–69	84	58	59	28	44	17
70–79	89	68	69	37	54	24
>80	93	76	78	47	65	32

FIGURE 3.3 Clinical pre-test probabilities[a] in patients with stable chest pain symptoms (From ESC guidelines (Ref. [14]) with permission). *ECG* electrocardiogram, *PTP* pre-test probability, *SCAD* stable coronary artery disease. [a]Probabilities of obstructive coronary disease shown reflect the estimates for patients aged 35, 45, 55, 65, 75 and 85 years. Groups in *white boxes* have a PTP <15 % and hence can be managed without further testing. Groups in *blue boxes* have a PTP of 15–65 %. They could have an exercise ECG if feasible as the initial test. However, if local expertise and availability permit a non-invasive imaging based test for ischaemia this would be preferable given the superior diagnostic capabilities of such tests. In young patients radiation issues should be considered. Groups in light red boxes have PTPs between 66 and 85 % and hence should have a non-invasive imaging functional test for making a diagnosis of SCAD. In groups in dark red boxes the PTP is >85 % and one can assume that SCAD is present. They need risk stratification only

enced by the prevalence of the disease in the population under study and the clinical features, including the presence of risk factors, present in a given individual [18].

ECG Stress Testing

In the absence of contraindications, and given its widespread availability and reduced cost, exercise ECG is recommended (recommendation level, I.B) as the initial test for establishing a diagnosis of ischaemic heart disease. This test is recommended in patients with chest pain suggestive of angina/myocardial ischaemia and intermediate PTP of coronary artery disease. Interestingly, despite the widespread use of different imaging modalities and the rapid growth of computerised tomographic angiography (CCTA) in the USA, current American guidelines for the assessment and management of stable angina specifically recommend stress testing as the initial diagnostic test of choice [1].

Stress Imaging for the Detection of Myocardial Ischaemia

There is little, if any, definitive evidence of superiority of one specific imaging modality over another, and none of these techniques have yet demonstrated improved clinical outcomes attributable to their diagnostic performance.

Stress Echocardiography

Stress echocardiography can be carried out using exercise (treadmill or bicycle-ergometer) or pharmacological agents as suitable stressors [19]. It is generally accepted that exercise provides a more physiological stimulus – such as that which usually triggers effort angina in patients- compared with pharmacological agents. In addition, data obtained during exercise, such as time to ischaemia, total exercise duration, maximum workload and blood pressure response, provide important data that can be useful for risk stratification. ESC guideline recommendations for the use of diagnostic exercise or pharmacological stress testing are shown in Fig. 3.4 (take from Table 15 in ESC guidelines). In patients who are unable to exercise, pharmacological agents, particularly dobutamine, represent an excellent alternative choice. A note of caution, however, as data on specificity and sensitivity of stress testing echocardiography mentioned in the ESC guidelines are probably not an accurate reflection of the improved diagnostic ability of more recent echocardiographic techniques, such as contrast echocardiography. The information used in the guidelines refers to inducible wall thickening abnormalities as a marker of ischaemia. Myocardial contrast echocardiography (microbubbles) provides information beyond wall thickening. The technique is not widely used currently [20, 21], but it is likely that we will see an increasing use of this methodology, as contrast stress echocardiography enhances image quality.

Myocardial Perfusion Scintigraphy (Single Photon Emission Computed Tomography SPECT)

SPECT perfusion scintigraphy allows the assessment of regional myocardial tracer uptake, to identify relative regional myocardial blood flow. Areas of myocardial hypoperfusion are characterised by reduced tracer uptake during stress, compared with uptake at rest. Technetium-99m (^{99m}Tc) radiopharmaceuticals are commonly used with SPECT stress testing nowadays, as these agents are associated with less radiation hazard compared with ^{201}Tl. Like stress echocardiography, SPECT can be used during exercise or with the injection of dobutamine. It has higher sensitivity and specificity compared with ECG stress testing. Figure 3.5 summarises sensitivity and specificity values for the different diagnostic myocardial perfusion techniques currently used in clinical practice.

Recommendations	Class[a]	Level[a]
An imaging stress test is recommended as the initial test for diagnosing SCAD if the PTP is between 66–85% or i LVEF is <50% in Patients without typical angina.	I	B
An imaging stress test is recommended in patients with resting ECG abnormalities which prevent accurate interpretation of ECG changes during stress.	I	B
Exercise stress testing is recommended rather then pharmacologic testing whenever possible.	I	C
An imaging stress test should be considered in symptomatic patients with prior revascularization (PCI or CABG).	IIa	B
An imaging stress test should be considered to assess the functional severity of intermediate lesions on coronary arteriography.	IIa	B

FIGURE 3.4 Use of exercise or pharmacologic stress testing in combination with imaging, as recommended by the ESC guidelines on management of angina (With permission). *CABG* coronary artery bypass graft, *ECG* electrocardiogram, *PCI* percutaneous coronary intervention, *PTP* pre-test probability, *SCAD* stable coronary artery disease. [a]Class of recommendation. [b]Level of evidence

	Diagnosis of CAD	
	Sensitivity (%)	Specificity (%)
Exercise ECG [a, 91, 94, 95]	45–50	85–90
Exercise stress echocardiography[96]	80–85	80–88
Exercise stress SPECT[96-99]	73–92	63–87
Dobutamine stress echocardiography[96]	79–83	82–86
Dobutamine stress MRI[b,100]	79–88	81–91
Vasodilator stress echocardiography[96]	72–79	92–95
Vasodilator stress SPECT[96, 99]	90–91	75–84
Vasodilator stress MRI[b, 98, 100-102]	67–94	61–85
Coronary CTA[c, 103, 105]	95–99	64–83
Vasodilator stress PET[97, 99, 106]	81–97	74–91

FIGURE 3.5 Sensitivity and specificity of tests commonly used to diagnose obstructive atherosclerotic coronary artery disease (From ESC guidelines, Ref. [14]). *CAD* coronary artery disease, *CTA* computed tomography angiography, *ECG* electrocardiogram, *MRI* magnetic resonance imaging, *PET* positron emission tomography, *SPECT* single photon emission computed tomography. [a]Results without/with minimal referral bias. [b]Results obtained in populations with medium-to-high prevalence of disease without compensation for referral bias. [c]Results obtained in populations with low-to-medium prevalence of disease

Positron Emission Tomography

Myocardial perfusion imaging, using positron emission tomography (PET), is superior to other imaging modalities particularly regarding its ability to quantify myocardial blood flow per gram of heart tissue (mL/min/g). This allows an accurate assessment of coronary flow reserve and the investigation of coronary microvascular disease [22]. Unfortunately, PET scanners are more expensive than SPECT scanners and therefore less readily available in clinical practice.

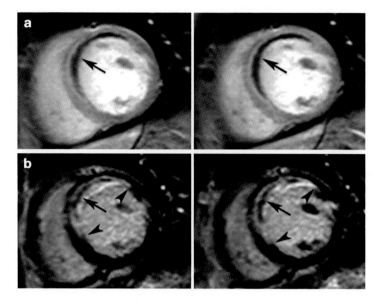

FIGURE 3.6 Cardiac MRI for the assessment of microvascular angina (From Bekkers et al. [67]). Cardiovascular MRI. A set of two corresponding short-axis images with a single breathhold 3-dimensional inversion recovery gradient-echo pulse sequence. (**a**) Early (2 min after contrast injection) contrast-enhanced cardiovascular magnetic resonance imaging (MRI) showing a central hypoenhanced area corresponding to microvascular obstruction (MVO) in the antero-septal region (*arrows*, early MVO). (**b**) Late gadolinium-enhanced cardiovascular MRI (10 min after contrast injection) showing hyperenhancement indicating an anteroseptal myocardial infarction (*arrowheads*) with a central zone of MVO (*arrows*, late MVO)

Stress Cardiac Magnetic Resonance

Cardiac magnetic resonance (CMR) stress testing is an excellent technique for the assessment of structural and functional heart abnormalities. CMR has been shown to have a safety profile comparable to that of dobutamine stress echocardiography [23, 24]. Perfusion CMR, using adenosine as an arteriolar vasodilator, is currently performed in tertiary centres for the assessment of subendocardial ischaemia and CFR in patients with suspected microvascular angina (Fig. 3.6).

Anatomical Diagnosis of Coronary Artery Disease

Coronary Computed Tomography Angiography (CCTA)

American guidelines [1] recommend CCTA for patients who are unable to undergo stress testing. It is conceivable however that as more evidence continues to accumulate regarding the usefulness of CCTA, this diagnostic modality will have a more prominent role in future diagnostic strategies. In patients with suspected CAD, studies using 64-slice CT have reported sensitivities of 95–99 % and specificities of 64–83 % (Fig. 3.5), as well as negative predictive values of 97–99 %, for the identification of individuals with at least one coronary artery stenosis as detected by invasive coronary arteriography [25, 26]. The presence of severe and extensive coronary calcification and also that of coronary stents reduce the diagnostic accuracy of coronary CCTA [27, 28]. The assessment of coronary artery bypass grafts is highly accurate while the evaluation of native coronary vessels in post-bypass patients has been reported to yield false positive findings [29, 30].

Further large prospective studies are required to establish the role of CCTA in patient risk stratification and prognosis. One such study, the SCOT-HEART study [31], aimed to assess the diagnostic utility of CCTA against findings at conventional invasive coronary angiography, and to investigate the timing and therapeutic implementation of CCTA-guided changes in preventive treatment. This was a prospective, open-label, parallel group, multicenter, randomized controlled trial that assessed the role of CCTA in patients with suspected angina due to coronary heart disease. 4,146 patients age 18–75 years were recruited from cardiology chest pain clinics where they were referred with suspected angina due to coronary heart disease. Participants were randomized 1:1 to standard care or standard care plus 64-slice CCTA. Invasive angiography was less likely to demonstrate normal coronary arteries (20 vs. 56; HR 0.39; 95 % CI 0.23–0.68; p < 0.001) but more likely to show obstructive coronary artery disease (283 vs. 230; HR: 1.29 [95 % CI: 1.08–1.55]; p = 0.005) in those allocated to CCTA. More preventative therapies (283 vs. 74; HR: 4.03 [95 % CI: 3.12–5.20]; p < 0.001) were initiated after CCTA, with each drug commencing at a median of 48–52 days after clinic attendance. From the median time for preventive therapy initiation (50 days), fatal and nonfatal myocardial infarction was halved in patients allocated to CCTA compared with those assigned to standard care (17 vs. 34; HR: 0.50 [95 % CI: 0.28–0.88]; p = 0.020). Cumulative 6-month costs were slightly higher with CCTA: difference $462 (95 % CI: $303–$621). The investigators concluded that in patients with suspected angina due to coronary heart disease, CCTA leads to more appropriate use of invasive angiography and alterations in preventive therapies that were associated with a halving of fatal and non-fatal myocardial infarction. If results in the SCOT-HEART [31] study are confirmed by other large trials, CCTA is likely to find a major role in diagnostic strategies for angina pectoris in the near future.

Conventional Invasive Angiography

Improved diagnostic accuracy and substantial reductions in complication rates in recent years make invasive coronary arteriography a suitable method to safely assess coronary anatomy as part of a comprehensive diagnostic strategy in patients with stable angina. The use of the radial artery for access has contributed to early hospital discharge and perambulation after the procedure [32]. The composite rate of major complications associated with femoral diagnostic angiography (mainly bleeding requiring blood transfusion) is less than 2 % [33], and the composite rate of death, MI, or stroke ranges from 0.1 to 0.2 % [34]. The ESC guidelines [14] recommend performing conventional angiography for the assessment of angina in patients with reduced LVEF, in patients who are unable to undergo functional testing and in subjects whose professions – due to statutory regulations – require specific assessment of coronary anatomy (i.e. airline pilots).

Patient Risk Stratification as Part of the Diagnostic Process

Conventional risk factors for coronary disease have been shown to have an adverse influence on prognosis, particularly in subjects who have already developed coronary artery disease. Key determinants of impaired clinical outcomes in subjects with coronary artery disease have been listed in Fig. 3.7 (from Table 17 ESC guidelines).

Interestingly, in recent years it has become apparent that an elevated resting heart rate is also a marker of worse long term prognosis in individuals with coronary artery disease [35, 36].

Recent large epidemiologic studies have confirmed earlier observations that resting heart rate is an independent predictor

Exercise stress ECG[b]	High risk	CV mortality >3 %/year.
	Intermediate risk	CV mortality between 1 and 3 %/year.
	Low risk	CV mortality <1 %/year.
Ischaemia imaging	High risk	Area of ischaemia >10 % (>10 % for SPECT; limited quantitative data for CMR – probably ≥2/16 segments with new perfusion defects or ≥3 dobutamine-induced dysfunctional segments; ≥3 segments of LV by stress echo).
	Intermediate risk	Area of ischaemia between 1 to 10% or any ischaemia less than high risk by CMR or stress echo.
	Low risk	No ischaemia.
Coronary CTA[c]	High risk	Significant lesions of high risk category (three-vessel disease with proximal stenoses, LM, and proximal anterior descending CAD).
	Intermediate risk	Significant lesion(s) in large and proximal coronary artery(ies) but not high risk category.
	Low risk	Normal coronary artery or plaques only.

FIGURE 3.7 Definitions of cardiovascular risk for various test modalities[a] (From Ref. [14] with permission). *CAD* coronary artery disease, *CMR* cardiac magnetic resonance, *CTA* computed tomography angiography, *CV* cardiovascular, *ECG* electrocardiogram, *ICA* invasive coronary angiography, *LM* left main, *PTP* pre-test probability, *SPECT* single photon emission computed tomography. [a]For detailed explanation on rationale for risk stratification scheme see web addenda. [b]From nomogram (see web addenda) or http://www.cardiology.org/tools/medcalc/duke/. Consider possible overestimation of presence of significant multivessel disease by coronary CTA in patients with high intermediate PTP (≥50 %) and/or severe diffuse or focal coronary calcifications and consider performing additional stress testing in patients without severe symptoms before ICA

of cardiovascular and all-cause mortality in men and women with and without cardiovascular disease. Clinical trial data suggest that heart rate reduction *per se* is an important mechanism of benefit of beta-blockers [37, 38] and other heart-rate lowering drugs such as ivabradine, used in chronic heart failure [39].

In stable angina pectoris, heart rate reductions with ivabradine resulted in antianginal effects but no improvement in clinical outcomes was documented [40].

Pathophysiological studies indicate that a relatively high HR has direct detrimental effects on the progression of coronary atherosclerosis, on the occurrence of myocardial ischemia and ventricular arrhythmias, and on left ventricular function. Although it may be difficult to define an optimal HR for a given individual, it seems desirable to maintain resting HR substantially below the traditionally defined tachycardia threshold of 90 or 100 beats/min [36].

The long-term prognosis of stable angina associated with coronary artery disease depends on: clinical and demographic variables, the presence of myocardial ischaemia at low workload on stress testing, baseline LV function, and severity of coronary disease as assessed angiographically. Patients with ischaemic heart disease are at increased risk of adverse events: particularly myocardial infarction, heart failure and cardiovascular death. The diagnostic strategies recommended by American and European guidelines allow for risk stratification of the patients who are under investigation for angina. This has practical value as, for example, patients requiring revascularisation can be identified in the process. The ESC guidelines [14] define "high risk" patients as those with an estimated annual mortality >3 % and these patients require myocardial revascularisaton. Patients at low risk of events have an annual mortality of 1 % per year, while the group considered to be at intermediate event risk has an annual mortality ≥1 % but ≤3 % per year.

Risk evaluation is based on the clinical assessment of the patient, their ventricular function, ischaemic and haemodynamic responses to stress testing and coronary anatomy, as assessed by angiography. Figure 3.7 (Taken from Table 17 ESC guidelines) summarises ESC criteria to define levels of risk depending on whether clinical evaluation, LV function or anatomical markers are used for risk assessment. Clinically accessible instruments based on basic parameters are also available that can help clinicians to risk stratify patients during the consultation [15].

A detailed clinical evaluation of the patient, including a baseline ECG and routine blood tests, often provide relevant prognostic information. Severe angina symptoms occurring at a low workload, history of previous myocardial infarction and heart failure represent important markers of impaired outcome [41–44]. The presence of conventional risk factors such as hypertension, smoking, hypercholesterolaemia, metabolic syndrome, diabetes mellitus, are predictors of impaired clinical outcome, particularly in patients with coronary artery disease [45]. Chronic kidney disease, chronic inflammatory conditions and peripheral vascular disease have become established risk factors for accelerated disease progression [46, 47].

Despite guidelines [14] that advocate the use of stress testing to risk assess patients with angina due to coronary artery disease, no randomised studies are available to endorse such a recommendation. Nevertheless, expert consensus at present is that low risk patients, as assessed clinically, with a normal response to exercise ECG stress testing, have a very good prognosis [48]. The Duke treadmill score (http://www.cardiology.org/tools/medcalc/duke/), which combines total exercise duration, ST-segment changes and the occurrence of angina during effort to calculate event risk [49], has been validated extensively and is used worldwide in both clinical practice and research protocols.

Stress testing using imaging modalities is useful for risk stratification. Stress echocardiography has good negative predictive value in subjects with no inducible regional wall motion abnormalities [50–52], and a good positive predictive value when wall motion abnormalities are detected in more than three of the conventional 17 LV segment model scheme (estimated annual mortality >3 %) [53–55]. Patients in this higher risk cohort should be considered for coronary arteriography with a view to offering revascularisation if appropriate.

Stress perfusion scintigraphy, whether using SPECT or PET, is useful for risk stratification. Large studies have reported that abnormal perfusion stress tests with large defects or evidence of LV dysfunction are predictors of poor clinical outcomes [55–57], while normal stress perfusion studies predict very low risk of cardiac death and myocardial infarction [58]. Studies using stress cardiac magnetic resonance have also shown an association between poor clinical prognosis and abnormal test results and, conversely, excellent prognosis with 99 % event-free survival in patients with no evidence of ischaemia during stress testing [59, 60]. Head-to-head comparisons in carefully selected populations are necessary to establish whether there are true differences regarding the predictive value of these different stress test imaging modalities.

Anatomical assessment of disease extent and severity has prognostic value, whether assessed by CCTA or invasive coronary angiography. Large prospective trials have documented the prognostic value of CCTA, even after controlling for risk factors [61–65]. Low risk of events rates were documented when no stenoses were detected and, conversely, increased annual mortality rates were found, similar to that in studies using conventional invasive coronary arteriography, in patients with CCTA left main stenosis or triple vessel disease [61, 66]. Invasive coronary angiography is – at present – the gold standard for the assessment of anatomic severity of atheromatous plaques and their role as prognostic indicators in patients with angina.

References

1. Fihn SD, Gardin JM, Abrams J, Berra K, Blankenship JC, Dallas AP, Douglas PS, Foody JM, Gerber TC, Hinderliter AL, King 3rd SB, Kligfield PD, Krumholz HM, Kwong RYK, Lim MJ,

Linderbaum JA, Mack MJ, Munger MA, Prager RL, Sabik JF, Shaw LJ, Sikkema JD, Smith CRJ, Smith SCJ, Spertus JA, Williams SV. 2012 ACCF/AHA/ACP/AATS/PCNA/SCAI/STS guideline for the diagnosis and management of patients with stable ischemic heart disease: a report of the American College of Cardiology Foundation/American Heart Association Task Force on Practice Guidelines, and the American College of Physicians, American Association for Thoracic Surgery, Preventive Cardiovascular Nurses Association, Society for Cardiovascular Angiography and Interventions, and Society of Thoracic Surgeons. J Am Coll Cardiol. 2012;60:e44–164.

2. Libby P, Theroux P. Pathophysiology of coronary artery disease. Circulation. 2005;111:3481–8.

3. Hansson GK. Inflammation, atherosclerosis, and coronary artery disease. N Engl J Med. 2005;352:1685–95.

4. Libby P. Inflammation in atherosclerosis. Arterioscler Thromb Vasc Biol. 2012;32:2045–51.

5. Bayturan O, Kapadia S, Nicholls SJ, Tuzcu EM, Shao M, Uno K, Shreevatsa A, Lavoie AJ, Wolski K, Schoenhagen P, Nissen SE. Clinical predictors of plaque progression despite very low levels of low-density lipoprotein cholesterol. J Am Coll Cardiol. 2010;55:2736–42.

6. Chhatriwalla AK, Nicholls SJ, Wang TH, Wolski K, Sipahi I, Crowe T, Schoenhagen P, Kapadia S, Tuzcu EM, Nissen SE. Low levels of low-density lipoprotein cholesterol and blood pressure and progression of coronary atherosclerosis. J Am Coll Cardiol. 2009;53:1110–5.

7. Kronmal RA, McClelland RL, Detrano R, Shea S, Lima JA, Cushman M, Bild DE, Burke GL. Risk factors for the progression of coronary artery calcification in asymptomatic subjects: results from the Multi-Ethnic Study of Atherosclerosis (MESA). Circulation. 2007;115:2722–30.

8. Nicholls SJ, Hsu A, Wolski K, Hu B, Bayturan O, Lavoie A, Uno K, Tuzcu EM, Nissen SE. Intravascular ultrasound-derived measures of coronary atherosclerotic plaque burden and clinical outcome. J Am Coll Cardiol. 2010;55:2399–407.

9. Pekkanen J, Linn S, Heiss G, Suchindran CM, Leon A, Rifkind BM, Tyroler HA. Ten-year mortality from cardiovascular disease in relation to cholesterol level among men with and without preexisting cardiovascular disease. N Engl J Med. 1990;322:1700–7.

10. Bayturan O, Tuzcu EM, Uno K, Lavoie AJ, Hu T, Shreevatsa A, Wolski K, Schoenhagen P, Kapadia S, Nissen SE, Nicholls SJ. Comparison of rates of progression of coronary atherosclerosis in patients with diabetes mellitus versus those with the metabolic syndrome. Am J Cardiol. 2010;105:1735–9.

11. Frey P, Waters DD, DeMicco DA, Breazna A, Samuels L, Pipe A, Wun C-C, Benowitz NL. Impact of smoking on cardiovascular events in patients with coronary disease receiving contemporary medical therapy (from the Treating to New Targets [TNT] and the Incremental Decrease in End Points Through Aggressive Lipid Lowering [IDEAL] trials). Am J Cardiol. 2011;107:145–50.

12. Otaki Y, Gransar H, Berman DS, Cheng VY, Dey D, Lin FY, Achenbach S, Al-Mallah M, Budoff MJ, Cademartiri F, Callister TQ, Chang H-J, Chinnaiyan K, Chow BJW, Delago A, Hadamitzky M, Hausleiter J, Kaufmann P, Maffei E, Raff G, Shaw LJ, Villines TC, Dunning A, Min JK. Impact of family history of coronary artery disease in young individuals (from the CONFIRM registry). Am J Cardiol. 2013;111:1081–6.

13. Nicholls SJ, Ballantyne CM, Barter PJ, Chapman MJ, Erbel RM, Libby P, Raichlen JS, Uno K, Borgman M, Wolski K, Nissen SE. Effect of two intensive statin regimens on progression of coronary disease. N Engl J Med. 2011;365:2078–87.

14. Montalescot G, Sechtem U, Achenbach S, Andreotti F, Arden C, Budaj A, Bugiardini R, Crea F, Cuisset T, Di Mario C, Ferreira JR, Gersh BJ, Gitt AK, Hulot J-S, Marx N, Opie LH, Pfisterer M, Prescott E, Ruschitzka F, Sabate M, Senior R, Taggart DP, van der Wall EE, Vrints CJM, Zamorano JL, Achenbach S, Baumgartner H, Bax JJ, Bueno H, Dean V, et al. 2013 ESC guidelines on the management of stable coronary artery disease: the Task Force on the management of stable coronary artery disease of the European Society of Cardiology. Eur Heart J. 2013;34:2949–3003.

15. Bosner S, Haasenritter J, Becker A, Karatolios K, Vaucher P, Gencer B, Herzig L, Heinzel-Gutenbrunner M, Schaefer JR, Abu Hani M, Keller H, Sonnichsen AC, Baum E, Donner-Banzhoff N. Ruling out coronary artery disease in primary care: development and validation of a simple prediction rule. CMAJ. 2010;182:1295–300.

16. Campeau L. Letter: grading of angina pectoris. Circulation. 1976;54:522–3.

17. Cohn PF, Fox KM, Daly C. Silent myocardial ischemia. Circulation. 2003;108:1263–77.
18. Diamond GA, Forrester JS. Analysis of probability as an aid in the clinical diagnosis of coronary-artery disease. N Engl J Med. 1979;300:1350–8.
19. Sicari R, Nihoyannopoulos P, Evangelista A, Kasprzak J, Lancellotti P, Poldermans D, Voigt J-U, Zamorano JL. Stress echocardiography expert consensus statement: European Association of Echocardiography (EAE) (a registered branch of the ESC). Eur J Echocardiogr. 2008;9:415–37.
20. Senior R, Becher H, Monaghan M, Agati L, Zamorano J, Vanoverschelde JL, Nihoyannopoulos P. Contrast echocardiography: evidence-based recommendations by European Association of Echocardiography. Eur J Echocardiogr. 2009;10:194–212.
21. Senior R, Moreo A, Gaibazzi N, Agati L, Tiemann K, Shivalkar B, von Bardeleben S, Galiuto L, Lardoux H, Trocino G, Carrio I, Le Guludec D, Sambuceti G, Becher H, Colonna P, Ten Cate F, Bramucci E, Cohen A, Bezante G, Aggeli C, Kasprzak JD. Comparison of sulfur hexafluoride microbubble (SonoVue)-enhanced myocardial contrast echocardiography with gated single-photon emission computed tomography for detection of significant coronary artery disease: a large European multi-center study. J Am Coll Cardiol. 2013;62:1353–61.
22. Kajander S, Joutsiniemi E, Saraste M, Pietila M, Ukkonen H, Saraste A, Sipila HT, Teras M, Maki M, Airaksinen J, Hartiala J, Knuuti J. Cardiac positron emission tomography/computed tomography imaging accurately detects anatomically and functionally significant coronary artery disease. Circulation. 2010;122:603–13.
23. Wahl A, Paetsch I, Gollesch A, Roethemeyer S, Foell D, Gebker R, Langreck H, Klein C, Fleck E, Nagel E. Safety and feasibility of high-dose dobutamine-atropine stress cardiovascular magnetic resonance for diagnosis of myocardial ischaemia: experience in 1000 consecutive cases. Eur Heart J. 2004;25:1230–6.
24. Secknus MA, Marwick TH. Evolution of dobutamine echocardiography protocols and indications: safety and side effects in 3,011 studies over 5 years. J Am Coll Cardiol. 1997;29:1234–40.
25. Budoff MJ, Dowe D, Jollis JG, Gitter M, Sutherland J, Halamert E, Scherer M, Bellinger R, Martin A, Benton R, Delago A, Min JK. Diagnostic performance of 64-multidetector row coronary computed tomographic angiography for evaluation of coronary

artery stenosis in individuals without known coronary artery disease: results from the prospective multicenter ACCURACY (Assessment by Coronary Computed Tomographic Angiography of Individuals Undergoing Invasive Coronary Angiography) trial. J Am Coll Cardiol. 2008;52:1724–32.

26. Meijboom WB, Meijs MFL, Schuijf JD, Cramer MJ, Mollet NR, van Mieghem CAG, Nieman K, van Werkhoven JM, Pundziute G, Weustink AC, de Vos AM, Pugliese F, Rensing B, Jukema JW, Bax JJ, Prokop M, Doevendans PA, Hunink MGM, Krestin GP, de Feyter PJ. Diagnostic accuracy of 64-slice computed tomography coronary angiography: a prospective, multicenter, multivendor study. J Am Coll Cardiol. 2008;52:2135–44.

27. Brodoefel H, Burgstahler C, Tsiflikas I, Reimann A, Schroeder S, Claussen CD, Heuschmid M, Kopp AF. Dual-source CT: effect of heart rate, heart rate variability, and calcification on image quality and diagnostic accuracy. Radiology. 2008;247:346–55.

28. Vavere AL, Arbab-Zadeh A, Rochitte CE, Dewey M, Niinuma H, Gottlieb I, Clouse ME, Bush DE, Hoe JWM, de Roos A, Cox C, Lima JAC, Miller JM. Coronary artery stenoses: accuracy of 64-detector row CT angiography in segments with mild, moderate, or severe calcification – a subanalysis of the CORE-64 trial. Radiology. 2011;261:100–8.

29. Ropers D, Pohle F-K, Kuettner A, Pflederer T, Anders K, Daniel WG, Bautz W, Baum U, Achenbach S. Diagnostic accuracy of noninvasive coronary angiography in patients after bypass surgery using 64-slice spiral computed tomography with 330-ms gantry rotation. Circulation. 2006;114:2334–41; quiz 2334.

30. Weustink AC, Nieman K, Pugliese F, Mollet NR, Meijboom WB, van Mieghem C, ten Kate G-J, Cademartiri F, Krestin GP, de Feyter PJ. Diagnostic accuracy of computed tomography angiography in patients after bypass grafting: comparison with invasive coronary angiography. JACC Cardiovasc Imaging. 2009;2:816–24.

31. Williams MC, Hunter A, Shah ASV, Assi V, Lewis S, Smith J, Berry C, Boon NA, Clark E, Flather M, Forbes J, McLean S, Roditi G, van Beek EJR, Timmis AD, Newby DE. Use of coronary computed tomographic angiography to guide management of patients with coronary disease. J Am Coll Cardiol. 2016;67:1759–68.

32. Jolly SS, Amlani S, Hamon M, Yusuf S, Mehta SR. Radial versus femoral access for coronary angiography or intervention and the impact on major bleeding and ischemic events: a systematic

review and meta-analysis of randomized trials. Am Heart J. 2009;157:132–40.

33. Arora N, Matheny ME, Sepke C, Resnic FS. A propensity analysis of the risk of vascular complications after cardiac catheterization procedures with the use of vascular closure devices. Am Heart J. 2007;153:606–11.

34. Noto TJJ, Johnson LW, Krone R, Weaver WF, Clark DA, Kramer JRJ, Vetrovec GW. Cardiac catheterization 1990: a report of the Registry of the Society for Cardiac Angiography and Interventions (SCA&I). Cathet Cardiovasc Diagn. 1991;24:75–83.

35. Diaz A, Bourassa MG, Guertin M-C, Tardif J-C. Long-term prognostic value of resting heart rate in patients with suspected or proven coronary artery disease. Eur Heart J. 2005;26:967–74.

36. Fox K, Borer JS, Camm AJ, Danchin N, Ferrari R, Lopez Sendon JL, Steg PG, Tardif J-C, Tavazzi L, Tendera M. Resting heart rate in cardiovascular disease. J Am Coll Cardiol. 2007;50:823–30.

37. Kjekshus JK. Importance of heart rate in determining beta-blocker efficacy in acute and long-term acute myocardial infarction intervention trials. Am J Cardiol. 1986;57:43F–9.

38. Gundersen T, Grottum P, Pedersen T, Kjekshus JK. Effect of timolol on mortality and reinfarction after acute myocardial infarction: prognostic importance of heart rate at rest. Am J Cardiol. 1986;58:20–4.

39. Swedberg K, Komajda M, Bohm M, Borer JS, Ford I, Dubost-Brama A, Lerebours G, Tavazzi L. Ivabradine and outcomes in chronic heart failure (SHIFT): a randomised placebo-controlled study. Lancet. 2010;376:875–85.

40. Fox K, Ford I, Steg PG, Tardif J-C, Tendera M, Ferrari R. Ivabradine in stable coronary artery disease without clinical heart failure. N Engl J Med. 2014;371:1091–9.

41. Weiner DA, Ryan TJ, McCabe CH, Chaitman BR, Sheffield LT, Ferguson JC, Fisher LD, Tristani F. Prognostic importance of a clinical profile and exercise test in medically treated patients with coronary artery disease. J Am Coll Cardiol. 1984;3:772–9.

42. Hammermeister KE, DeRouen TA, Dodge HT. Variables predictive of survival in patients with coronary disease. Selection by univariate and multivariate analyses from the clinical, electro-cardiographic, exercise, arteriographic, and quantitative angiographic evaluations. Circulation. 1979;59:421–30.

43. Califf RM, Mark DB, Harrell FEJ, Hlatky MA, Lee KL, Rosati RA, Pryor DB. Importance of clinical measures of ischemia in

the prognosis of patients with documented coronary artery disease. J Am Coll Cardiol. 1988;11:20–6.

44. Pryor DB, Shaw L, McCants CB, Lee KL, Mark DB, Harrell FEJ, Muhlbaier LH, Califf RM. Value of the history and physical in identifying patients at increased risk for coronary artery disease. Ann Intern Med. 1993;118:81–90.

45. Hjemdahl P, Eriksson SV, Held C, Forslund L, Nasman P, Rehnqvist N. Favourable long term prognosis in stable angina pectoris: an extended follow up of the angina prognosis study in Stockholm (APSIS). Heart. 2006;92:177–82.

46. Di Angelantonio E, Chowdhury R, Sarwar N, Aspelund T, Danesh J, Gudnason V. Chronic kidney disease and risk of major cardiovascular disease and non-vascular mortality: prospective population based cohort study. BMJ. 2010;341:c4986.

47. Wilson PWF, D'Agostino RS, Bhatt DL, Eagle K, Pencina MJ, Smith SC, Alberts MJ, Dallongeville J, Goto S, Hirsch AT, Liau C-S, Ohman EM, Rother J, Reid C, Mas J-L, Steg PG. An international model to predict recurrent cardiovascular disease. Am J Med. 2012;125:695–703.e1.

48. Miller TD, Roger VL, Hodge DO, Gibbons RJ. A simple clinical score accurately predicts outcome in a community-based population undergoing stress testing. Am J Med. 2005;118:866–72.

49. Mark DB, Shaw L, Harrell FEJ, Hlatky MA, Lee KL, Bengtson JR, McCants CB, Califf RM, Pryor DB. Prognostic value of a treadmill exercise score in outpatients with suspected coronary artery disease. N Engl J Med. 1991;325:849–53.

50. Schinkel AFL, Bax JJ, Geleijnse ML, Boersma E, Elhendy A, Roelandt JRTC, Poldermans D. Noninvasive evaluation of ischaemic heart disease: myocardial perfusion imaging or stress echocardiography? Eur Heart J. 2003;24:789–800.

51. Marwick TH, Mehta R, Arheart K, Lauer MS. Use of exercise echocardiography for prognostic evaluation of patients with known or suspected coronary artery disease. J Am Coll Cardiol. 1997;30:83–90.

52. Olmos LI, Dakik H, Gordon R, Dunn JK, Verani MS, Quinones MA, Zoghbi WA. Long-term prognostic value of exercise echocardiography compared with exercise 201Tl, ECG, and clinical variables in patients evaluated for coronary artery disease. Circulation. 1998;98:2679–86.

53. Chelliah R, Anantharam B, Burden L, Alhajiri A, Senior R. Independent and incremental value of stress echocardiography over clinical and stress electrocardiographic parameters for

the prediction of hard cardiac events in new-onset suspected angina with no history of coronary artery disease. Eur J Echocardiogr. 2010;11:875–82.

54. Marwick TH, Case C, Vasey C, Allen S, Short L, Thomas JD. Prediction of mortality by exercise echocardiography: a strategy for combination with the duke treadmill score. Circulation. 2001;103:2566–71.

55. Lin FY, Dunning AM, Narula J, Shaw LJ, Gransar H, Berman DS, Min JK. Impact of an automated multimodality point-of-order decision support tool on rates of appropriate testing and clinical decision making for individuals with suspected coronary artery disease: a prospective multicenter study. J Am Coll Cardiol. 2013;62:308–16.

56. Hachamovitch R, Berman DS, Shaw LJ, Kiat H, Cohen I, Cabico JA, Friedman J, Diamond GA. Incremental prognostic value of myocardial perfusion single photon emission computed tomography for the prediction of cardiac death: differential stratification for risk of cardiac death and myocardial infarction. Circulation. 1998;97:535–43.

57. Hachamovitch R, Hayes SW, Friedman JD, Cohen I, Berman DS. Comparison of the short-term survival benefit associated with revascularization compared with medical therapy in patients with no prior coronary artery disease undergoing stress myocardial perfusion single photon emission computed tomography. Circulation. 2003;107:2900–7.

58. Brown KA. Prognostic value of thallium-201 myocardial perfusion imaging. A diagnostic tool comes of age. Circulation. 1991;83:363–81.

59. Korosoglou G, Elhmidi Y, Steen H, Schellberg D, Riedle N, Ahrens J, Lehrke S, Merten C, Lossnitzer D, Radeleff J, Zugck C, Giannitsis E, Katus HA. Prognostic value of high-dose dobutamine stress magnetic resonance imaging in 1,493 consecutive patients: assessment of myocardial wall motion and perfusion. J Am Coll Cardiol. 2010;56:1225–34.

60. Jahnke C, Nagel E, Gebker R, Kokocinski T, Kelle S, Manka R, Fleck E, Paetsch I. Prognostic value of cardiac magnetic resonance stress tests: adenosine stress perfusion and dobutamine stress wall motion imaging. Circulation. 2007;115:1769–76.

61. Min JK, Dunning A, Lin FY, Achenbach S, Al-Mallah M, Budoff MJ, Cademartiri F, Callister TQ, Chang H-J, Cheng V, Chinnaiyan K, Chow BJW, Delago A, Hadamitzky M, Hausleiter J, Kaufmann

P, Maffei E, Raff G, Shaw LJ, Villines T, Berman DS. Age- and sex-related differences in all-cause mortality risk based on coronary computed tomography angiography findings results from the International Multicenter CONFIRM (Coronary CT Angiography Evaluation for Clinical Outcomes: an International Multicenter Registry) of 23,854 patients without known coronary artery disease. J Am Coll Cardiol. 2011;58:849–60.

62. Hadamitzky M, Freissmuth B, Meyer T, Hein F, Kastrati A, Martinoff S, Schomig A, Hausleiter J. Prognostic value of coronary computed tomographic angiography for prediction of cardiac events in patients with suspected coronary artery disease. JACC Cardiovasc Imaging. 2009;2:404–11.

63. Chow BJW, Small G, Yam Y, Chen L, Achenbach S, Al-Mallah M, Berman DS, Budoff MJ, Cademartiri F, Callister TQ, Chang H-J, Cheng V, Chinnaiyan KM, Delago A, Dunning A, Hadamitzky M, Hausleiter J, Kaufmann P, Lin F, Maffei E, Raff GL, Shaw LJ, Villines TC, Min JK. Incremental prognostic value of cardiac computed tomography in coronary artery disease using CONFIRM: COroNary computed tomography angiography evaluation for clinical outcomes: an InteRnational Multicenter registry. Circ Cardiovasc Imaging. 2011;4:463–72.

64. Ostrom MP, Gopal A, Ahmadi N, Nasir K, Yang E, Kakadiaris I, Flores F, Mao SS, Budoff MJ. Mortality incidence and the severity of coronary atherosclerosis assessed by computed tomography angiography. J Am Coll Cardiol. 2008;52:1335–43.

65. Hulten EA, Carbonaro S, Petrillo SP, Mitchell JD, Villines TC. Prognostic value of cardiac computed tomography angiography: a systematic review and meta-analysis. J Am Coll Cardiol. 2011;57:1237–47.

66. Califf RM, Armstrong PW, Carver JR, D'Agostino RB, Strauss WE. 27th Bethesda Conference: matching the intensity of risk factor management with the hazard for coronary disease events. Task Force 5. Stratification of patients into high, medium and low risk subgroups for purposes of risk factor management. J Am Coll Cardiol. 1996;27:1007–19.

67. Bekkers SCAM, Yazdani SK, Virmani R, Waltenberger J. Microvascular obstruction: underlying pathophysiology and clinical diagnosis. J Am Coll Cardiol. 2010;55(16):1649–60. doi:10.1016/j.jacc.2009.12.037.

Chapter 4
Microvascular Angina: Diagnosis, Prognosis and Treatment

Abstract The term 'microvascular angina', proposed in the late 1980s, defines patients presenting with symptoms and signs of myocardial ischaemia, despite the presence of angiographically normal coronary arteries. Over the past few decades, evidence has accumulated that indicates the importance of coronary microcirculation abnormalities in the production of myocardial ischemia. Angina pectoris resulting from microvascular abnormalities, in the absence of flow limiting epicardial coronary artery stenoses, is well represented by the name "microvascular angina" (MVA). In patients with angina pectoris but without flow limiting coronary artery disease, MVA has been suggested to be the cause of symptoms and electrocardiographic changes indicative of myocardial ischaemia. MVA that occurs in patients with no cardiovascular or systemic conditions is known as "primary MVA" whereas MVA that occurs in the setting of specific diseases and/or conventional risk factors for coronary artery disease is defined as "secondary MVA". Both functional and structural abnormalities can affect the coronary microcirculation and lead to MVA. This chapter discusses the clinical importance, diagnosis and mechanisms of this intriguing condition.

J.C. Kaski, *Essentials in Stable Angina Pectoris*,
DOI 10.1007/978-3-319-41180-4_4,
© Springer International Publishing Switzerland 2016

As confirmed in recent clinical studies, over 50 % of patients undergoing coronary angiography with signs and/or symptoms of myocardial ischaemia are found to have normal or 'near normal' (non-obstructed) coronary arteries [1, 2]. Even after excluding non-cardiac causes of chest pain and Prinzmetal's variant angina, patients with angina and normal coronary arteriograms represent a heterogeneous group of patients, in whom different causes and pathophysiological mechanisms trigger coronary microvascular dysfunction (CMVD). The non-specific terms "chest pain with normal coronary arteries" and "cardiac syndrome X" have been used for many decades now, but do not provide a clear description of the mechanisms responsible for myocardial ischaemia in these patients [3, 4].

The term 'microvascular angina' was proposed in the late 1980s in an effort to define the underlying functional abnormality in patients presenting with chest pain and normal coronary arteries [5]. Over the past few decades, evidence has been gathered that implicates coronary microcirculation abnormalities in myocardial ischemia, via significant blood flow reduction in the absence of epicardial coronary artery obstructions. Angina pectoris resulting from microvascular abnormalities, in the absence of flow limiting epicardial coronary artery disease, is better reflected by the name "microvascular angina" (MVA), a term coined by Cannon and Epstein in 1988 [6]. Several comprehensive reviews have been published recently, which cover different aspects of this important topic [7–10]. In patients with angina pectoris but without flow limiting coronary artery disease, MVA has been suggested to be the cause of symptoms and electrocardiographic changes indicative of myocardial ischaemia. MVA that occurs in patients with no cardiovascular or systemic conditions is known as "primary MVA" whereas MVA that occurs in the setting of specific diseases and/or conventional risk factors for coronary artery disease is defined as "secondary MVA," as proposed by Lanza and Crea [7].

In 2007 Camici and Crea [11] proposed a classification of coronary microvascular dysfunction (CMVD) based on the

CMVD	Definition
Type 1	Primary, i.e. in the absence of structural heart disease
Type 2	In the presence of cardiomyopathies (incl, LVH, HCM, DCM, amyloidosis)
Type 3	In the presence of obstructive CAD (incl. ACS)
Type 4	After coronary interventions
Type 5	After cardiac transplantation
Modifiers	
Duration	Acute or chronic
Symptoms	Asymptomatic or symptomatic
Therapy	None, minimal, moderate, or maximal level

FIGURE 4.1 Modified clinical classification of coronary microvascular dysfunction (From Ref. [8], with permission). *ACS* acute coronary syndrome, *DCM* dilated cardiomyopathy, *HCM* hypertrophic cardiomyopathy, *LVH* left ventricular hypertrophy

clinical setting in which the condition develops, i.e. in patients with obstructive coronary artery disease, cardiomyopathy, systemic diseases, post revascularisation, etc.

In agreement with this approach, Herrmann et al. [8] proposed an additional subtype of MVA, i.e. CMVD post cardiac transplantation: mediated by alterations in autonomic tone, inflammation and immune mechanisms, and, possibly, defective endothelial progenitor cell recruitment (Fig. 4.1).

Clinical Presentation and Diagnosis

The main clinical consequence of the inability of the microvessels to increase blood flow sufficiently to match an increased myocardial oxygen demand is myocardial ischaemia. This resembles transient myocardial ischaemia resulting from flow-limiting epicardial stenoses, hence patients with CMVD often present with chronic stable angina and/or dyspnoea.

There are, however, differences regarding the blood flow limitation observed in MVA compared with that of obstructive coronary artery disease, and its impact on ventricular function as well as clinical presentation. In patients with coronary disease and flow limiting stenosis, blood flow reductions occur in the territory supplied by the stenotic vessel and result in segmental impairment of contractile function.

In contrast, in patients with CMVD, the abnormality in vascular function may affect different territories in a scattered fashion, as suggested by Maseri et al. [4] The subendocardial region of the left ventricle is commonly affected in patients with MVA [12]. These differences in myocardial perfusion abnormalities can explain why, until the advent of more accurate methods such as positron emission tomography and perfusion MRI, objective evidence of myocardial ischemia could not be obtained in most MVA patients with use of standard diagnostic techniques [7]. The above mentioned differences can also explain the diverse clinical presentations of MVA, and some of the differences between stable angina caused by stenosed epicardial coronary arteries and MVA.

Although angina symptoms are often indistinguishable from those caused by obstructive CAD, in MVA the chest pain can be long lasting and often show a relatively poor response to the administration of sublingual nitroglycerin [13, 14]. Another important clinical difference with classical stable angina caused by obstructive coronary disease is that MVA patients often present with both exertional and rest angina. The latter can be a predominant feature in some patients, and microvascular coronary artery spasm has to be investigated in these individuals [15].

Coronary microvascular spasm differs from typical Prinzmetal's variant angina in several aspects but it is often difficult – based on just clinical grounds – to establish a clear distinction between these two conditions. A history of rest angina is usually present in both patients with epicardial spasm and those with microvascular spasm. ST segment elevation, the hallmark of Prinzmetal's variant angina, can be also observed in patients with microvascular spasm.

Microvascular spasm in MVA patients is rarely associated with ST segment elevation, and commonly triggers chest pain and ST segment depression [15].

While symptoms are fully and rapidly relieved by sublingual nitrates in patients with epicardial coronary spasm, these agents tend to be less effective in MVA. Indeed, it has been reported that nitroglycerin may not provide quick and/or sufficient chest pain control in microvascular angina, compared with Prinzmetal's variant angina, as the small arterioles can forgo the vasodilatory effect of nitroglycerin [16]. If associated with severe hypotension, nitrates, per se, may cause angina. Epicardial vasospastic angina and MVA may coexist in some patients, suggesting a continuum of vascular dysfunction [17].

Diagnostic Techniques (Fig. 4.2)

Documentation of abnormal coronary microvascular responses to functional testing with the reproduction of symptoms is of central significance for this diagnosis [18]. Exercise ECG stress testing often triggers angina and typical ST-segment depression. Myocardial perfusion abnormalities are also relatively common in MVA, but the pattern of perfusion defects tends to be "patchy". Of interest, the absence of left ventricular contractile abnormalities, despite angina and ECG changes during echocardiographic stress testing, has been considered to strongly suggest MVA [19, 20].

More recently, probably due to more advanced echocardiographic technology, contractile abnormalities are detected in a larger proportion of MVA cases. Magnetic resonance imaging (MRI) can also outline microvascular obstruction albeit indirectly and with relatively low resolution [21].

Of importance, CMVD often results from functional and not necessarily structural abnormalities, or represents a combination of both mechanisms.

Consistent with the primary haemodynamic function of the coronary microcirculation, functional techniques (Fig. 4.2) for the assessment of the coronary microvasculature rely on

Method	Tracer	Primary parameter	Secondary parameter	Microvascular distinction	Endothelial assessment	Pros	Cons
PET	Radioisotopes	MBF (0.6–1.3mL/min/g)	MBF reserve (>2–2.5)	No	No	Validated and reproducibility	Limited availability, radioactivity
SPECT	Radioisotopes	Perfusion (no defect)	(Perfusion reserve)	No	No	Availbility, low costs	MBF only with dynamic upgrade, radioactivity
MDCT	Iodine contrast	MBF (0.9–1.3mL/min/g)	MBF reserve (>2–2.5)	No	No	Availbility	Investigational, image quality radiation
MRI	Gadolinium	MBF (0.7–1.1mL/min/g)	MBF reserve (>2–2.5)	No	No	One-stop test, no radiation or radioactivity	Investigational, technical limitations
MCE	Echo contrast	Perfusion, MBF option (0.5–2.9mL/min/g)	MBF reserve option (>2–2.5)	No	No	One-stop test, no radiation or radioactivity	Volumetric modelling, image quality
Doppler echo	Echo contrast	Flow velocity (24–36 cm/s)	Flow reserve (>2–2.5)	No	No	One-stop test, no radiation or radioactivity	No MBF option, position and image dependent
TFC	Iodine contrast	Contrast flow velocity (18–24)	TFC reserve (>2–2.5)	Assumed if no epicardial dx	No	Ease of use, low cost	No CBF option, subjectivity
MBG	Iodine contrast	Contrast staining (Grade 3)	None	Assumed if no epicardial dx	No	Ease of use, low cost	No CBF option, subjectivity
ICD	None	Flow velocity (10–22 cm/s)	(relative) flow velocity reserve	Assumed if no epicardial dx	Yes	Direct measurement	No CBF option, invasiveness
ICD+QCA/IVUS	Iodine contrast	CBF (44–59 mL/min)	CBF reserve (>2–2.5)	Yes	Yes	Complete assessment	Costs, invasiveness
TPS	Saline	IMF (15–22 U)	None	Yes	Yes	Complete assessment	Costs, invasiveness

PET, poistron emission tomography; SPECT, single photo emission computed tomography; MDCT, multi-detector computed tomography; MRI, magnetic resonance imaging; MCE, myocardial contrast echocardiography; TFC, TIMI frame cont; MBG, myocardial blush grade; ICD, intracoronary Doppler; QCA, quantitative coronary angiography; IVUS, intravascular ultrasound; TPS, temperature and pressure sensor; MBF, myocardial blood flow (mL/time/myocardial mass); CBF, coronary blood flow (mL/time unit).

Figure 4.2 Modalities to assess coronary microvascular function (From Ref. [8] with permission). *PET* poistron emission tomography, *SPECT* single photo emission computed tomography, *MDCT* multi-detector computed tomography, *MRI* magnetic resonance imaging, *MCE* myocardial contrast echocardiography, *TFC* TIMI frame count, *MBG* myocardial blush grade, *ICD* intracoronary Doppler, *QCA* quantitative coronary angiography, *IVUS* intravascular ultrasound, *TPS* temperature and pressure sensor, *MBF* myocardial blood flow (mL/time/myocardial mass), *CBF* cornary blood flow (mL/time unit)

the measurement of coronary blood flow reserve that is affected by alterations in vascular tone [22].

Positron emission tomography (PET) is the most established non-invasive technique for the assessment of CBF, as it allows the measurement of absolute regional myocardial blood flow (MBF) at rest and in response to various stimuli. Importantly, however, PET may lack sensitivity and specificity for the diagnosis of coronary vasomotor dysfunction [2, 23].

The most definitive evaluation of the coronary microcirculation remains invasive in nature. Simple angiographic techniques, such a TIMI frame count, can provide an approximate estimation of epicardial versus microvascular mechanisms [24].

Pressure – temperature sensor-tipped guidewires are available for the routine assessment of fractional flow reserve (FFR, by coronary pressure), coronary flow reserve (CFR, by coronary thermodilution) and calculation of the index of microvascular resistance (IMR) [25–27]. IMR is defined as the distal coronary pressure divided by the inverse of the hyperaemic mean transit time [26, 27]. This index was validated in experimental models but has several limitations. For instance, it is necessary to incorporate the collateral blood flow in the calculations, as otherwise IMR progressively increases with increasing degrees of epicardial coronary artery stenoses [26, 28].

As reviewed by Herrmann et al. [8], the functional status of the coronary microcirculation can be assessed by testing endothelium-dependent and endothelium-independent vascular responses [29]. Adenosine, dipyridamole, and papaverine are often used to trigger arteriolar vasodilation, and hence increase CBF, mainly by a direct relaxing effect on vascular smooth muscle cells. Thus, these agents are not suitable for the assessment of endothelium-dependent coronary microcirculation abnormalities [27].

Classically, intracoronary acetylcholine (ACH) has been used as a sensitive and safe test for the assessment of coronary vasomotor function in the catheterization laboratory. Its administration causes vasodilation under physiological conditions but, in the absence of a functional endothelium, it leads to vasoconstriction by the unopposed stimulation of muscarinic receptors on vascular smooth muscle cells [15, 29].

Bradykinin and substance-P are also suitable to test endothelial dependent vasomotor responses and, like ACH, also elicit a rapid vascular response [30].

Prognosis

Early studies in patients with chest pain and normal coronary arteriograms, usually encompassed under the term "cardiac syndrome X", suggested a benign long term prognosis in these patients [13, 31–34].

Among women with persistent signs and symptoms of ischaemia, microvascular dysfunction is associated with a relatively higher proportion of adverse events including heart failure and, to a lesser extent, myocardial infarction or increased mortality. Data from the NIH-NHLBI-sponsored Women's Ischemia Syndrome Evaluation (WISE) and related studies implicate adverse outcomes in relation to CMVD. Regardless of the presence or absence of epicardial disease – and even considering patients with normal coronary arteries – CMVD represents a marker of increased risk during long term follow up [35, 36].

The event-free survival, considering index events such as death, stroke, and hospitalization for heart failure, diverged more strongly after 4 years of follow up. In an unselected population of patients undergoing PET perfusion imaging, an adenosine CFR <2 provided additional prognostic information regarding cardiac death. Abnormal CRF was the most potent independent predictor of mortality [37].

In another study, an abnormal MBF response to cold pressure testing predicted a six to eight times higher incidence of ACS and need for revascularization during long-term follow-up, even in patients with normal coronaries on angiography [38].

A study by Murthy et al. [39] has extended observations in the WISE programme to men. They investigated 405 men and 813 women who were referred for evaluation of suspected coronary artery disease, with no previous history of coronary artery disease, and no visual evidence of coronary artery disease on rest/stress positron emission tomography myocardial perfusion imaging. Coronary flow reserve <2.0 was used to define the presence of coronary microvascular dysfunction (CMD). CMD was highly prevalent both in men and women (51 % and 54 %, respectively). The authors summarized their findings as follow: Major adverse cardiac events, including cardiac death, nonfatal myocardial infarction, late revascularization, and hospitalization for heart failure, were assessed in a blinded fashion over a median follow-up of 1.3 years (interquartile range, 0.5–2.3 years). Regardless of gender, coronary flow reserve was a powerful incremental predictor of major adverse cardiac events (hazard ratio, 0.80 [95 % confidence interval, 0.75–086] per 10 % increase in coronary flow reserve; $P < 0.0001$), and resulted in favorable net reclassification improvement (0.280 [95 % confidence interval, 0.049–0.512]) after adjustment for clinical risk and ventricular function. In a subgroup (n = 404; 307 women/97 men) without evidence of coronary artery calcification on gated computed tomography imaging, CMD was common in both sexes, despite normal stress perfusion imaging and no coronary artery calcification (44 % of men versus 48 % of women; Fisher exact test $P = 0.56$; equivalence $P = 0.041$). These results indicate that CMD is highly prevalent among at-risk individuals and is associated with adverse outcomes, regardless of gender. The high prevalence of CMD in both sexes suggests that CMD may be a useful target for future therapeutic interventions (Fig. 4.3).

A large epidemiological study by Jespersen et al. [40] provided important prognostic information in both men and women. This was the first study demonstrating that both men and women suspected of stable angina pectoris, and categorised with either normal coronary arteries or diffuse non-obstructive CAD, have increased risks of cardiovascular disease outcomes compared with a background population without known ischaemic heart disease, even

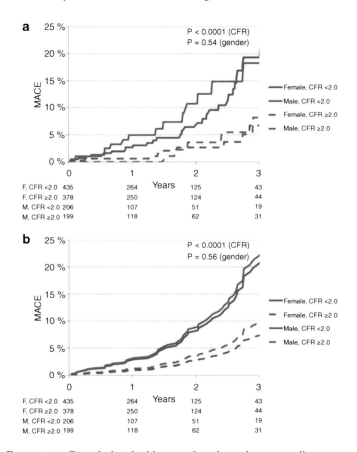

Figure 4.3 Cumulative incidence of major adverse cardiac events (MACEs) by sex and coronary flow reserve. Unadjusted (panel **a**) and adjusted (panel **b**) cumulative rate of MACEs by sex and coronary flow reserve (CFR) are presented in this figure. Data in panel **b** are adjusted for both the modified Duke clinical risk score and rest left ventricular ejection fraction (LVEF) (From Ref. [39] with permission)

after controlling for traditional cardiac risk factors and cardiac co-morbidity. In the period comprised between 1998 and 2009 they assessed 11,223 patients with stable angina pectoris referred for coronary angiography and

5705 participants from the Copenhagen City Heart Study, which acted as a control group. Main outcome measures were major adverse cardiovascular events (MACE), which included cardiovascular death, myocardial infarction, stroke or heart failure, and all-cause mortality. Significantly more women (65 %) than men (32 %) had no obstructive coronary artery disease (P < 0.001). In Cox's models adjusted for age, body mass index, diabetes, smoking, and use of lipid-lowering or antihypertensive medication, hazard ratios (HRs) associated with no obstructive coronary disease were similar in men and women. In the pooled analysis, the risk of MACE increased with increasing degrees of coronary artery disease with multivariable-adjusted HRs of 1.52 (95 % confidence interval, 1.27–1.83) for patients with normal coronary arteries and 1.85 (1.51–2.28) for patients with diffuse non-obstructive coronary artery disease, compared with the control population. For all-cause mortality, normal coronary arteries and diffuse non-obstructive CAD were associated with HRs of 1.29 (1.07–1.56) and 1.52 (1.24–1.88), respectively. The study thus showed that patients with stable angina and normal coronary arteries or diffuse non-obstructive coronary artery disease have elevated risks of MACE and all-cause mortality compared with a reference population without ischaemic heart disease (Fig. 4.4).

Although these latter studies have shed light on the changing prognostic pattern in patients with MVA, it is important to remember that most of these studies, particularly the earlier ones, have included heterogeneous patient groups. Lumping together patients with effort-induced angina, and completely normal coronary angiograms, with patients presenting with acute chest pain, coronary artery stenoses ranging from 20 to 50 %, impaired LV function, different comorbidities and conduction disturbances, is likely to confuse the issue. Large prospective studies are required to define very specifically which patient subgroups are at an increased risk of coronary events.

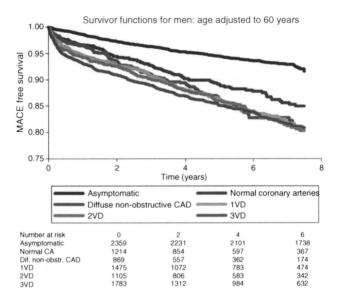

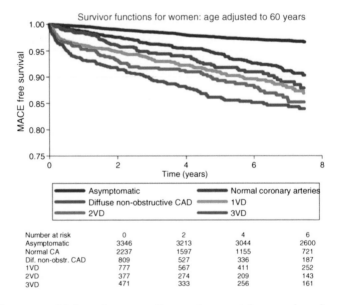

FIGURE 4.4 Major adverse cardiovascular event-free survivor functions for men and women. Age adjusted to 60 years. *VD* vessel disease (indicates ≥50 % stenosis) (From Ref. [40] with permission)

Treatment of Microvascular Angina

This topic has been recently reviewed by Lanza et al. [41] An important initial therapeutic measure in all patients with MVA is to treat coronary artery disease risk factors aggressively. Identifying the prevailing underlying mechanism is of paramount importance as this may give physicians the possibility of devising rational therapeutic strategies. Symptomatic treatment is currently based on results of small trials with little, if any, evidence base. Data from therapeutic trials available at present hardly represent conclusive evidence given the heterogeneous populations studied, variable patient selection criteria, small sample sizes, and lack of hard end points in most trials. Guidelines offer little if any help at present albeit the ESC guidelines have included some relevant information and conventional anti-ischaemic agents have been recommended as first line treatment. However, traditional antianginal drugs are effective in only approximately 50 % of MVA patients.

Short-acting nitrates can be used to treat anginal attacks, but they have been shown to be only partially effective in MVA [7].

Beta-blockers represent a rational approach in patients with effort-related angina, particularly if there is evidence of increased adrenergic activity (e.g. high heart rate at rest or at a low-workload). Beta-blockers are considered first line therapy by several investigators [7].

Calcium channel blockers have shown variable results in clinical trials but are widely used in MVA, as they have been reported to reduce angina episodes in most studies [42–44], albeit not in all [45]. Beneficial effects have been reported on exercise-induced angina and ST-segment depression [42–44, 46–48]. Calcium antagonist should be considered first-line therapy in patients with variable threshold effort angina [42] and patients with microvascular or epicardial coronary artery spasm.

Similarly, vasospastic angina and MVA can also be successfully treated with nitrates and with another vasodilator agent, nicorandil [49, 50]. However, recent data from the

Japanese coronary spasm association registry indicates a potentially higher incidence of major adverse cardiac events (MACE) when these two drugs are used together for treatment of chronic vasospastic angina [51].

Nitrates are not so effective in MVA due to the relatively small vasodilatory effect of these agents on small resistance vessels [52]. In clinical practice, however, they are useful in roughly 50 % of patients. Nicorandil has a more pronounced effect on the coronary microcirculation than nitrates, and therefore might be better suited for patients with microvascular angina, including those with microvascular spasm [53–55].

Improvement in exercise capacity has been observed in a small trial with nicorandil [56]. Nicorandil has direct dilator effects on coronary resistance vessels due to adenosine triphosphate (ATP) potassium channel opening and nitrate-like effects. Nicorandil has been shown to improve symptoms, myocardial perfusion, and signs of myocardial ischemia in MVA patients [53, 56]. This agent, when available, should be taken into account as a potentially useful vasodilator with cardioprotective effects. A limitation for the use of this drug are its side effects, particularly hypotension and – albeit less frequent – gut ulceration, as mentioned in other chapters of this book.

ACE inhibitors improve coronary microvascular function in patients with MVA by counteracting the vasoconstrictor effects of angiotensin II. These agents have been shown in small studies to improve symptoms and exercise capacity in MVA patients. ACE inhibitors may be helpful, particularly in MVA patients with hypertension and/or diabetes mellitus. ACE inhibitors might improve MVA through several effects, including microvascular dilatation, reduced oxidative stress, increased availability of nitric oxide and modulation of sympathetic nervous system activity related to the reduction of serum and tissue angiotensin II. Beneficial effects on anginal symptoms have been reported in small randomized controlled trials with ramipril, alone [43] or in combination with atorvastatin [57], and quinapril has also been reported to improve angina status in a more heterogeneous population of women with normal coronary arteries and <50 % coronary artery stenosis [58]. Furthermore, in other studies, ACE inhibitors were found to increase exercise tolerance [59, 60] and coronary microvascular function [61].

Alpha adrenergic antagonists may decrease vasoconstriction and may be considered in individual patients [62–64].

Small studies have reported beneficial effects with statins [65] and with oestrogen replacement treatment [66].

A significant number of patients with stable MVA are peri- or post-menopausal women [13], which suggest that oestrogen deficiency can play a pathogenic role. Indeed, oestrogen deficiency is associated with impaired endothelial function and increased adrenergic activity, typically present in MVA patients [67, 68]. Transdermal 17-beta-estradiol was shown to reduce angina episodes in post-menopausal women with MVA in a placebo-controlled cross-over study [69], and to improve exercise-induced angina and ST-segment depression in another study [66]. Thus, oestrogens can be helpful in the management of peri-menopausal women with MVA, although the initial benefits may decrease over long-term treatment [70]; furthermore, it is necessary to address safety concerns regarding the long-term administration of oestrogen [71].

It has been suggested that patients with angina refractory to the medications mentioned in this section may benefits from other forms of treatment. Xanthine derivatives (aminophylline, bamiphylline) can be added to the anti-ischaemic treatment to try to reduce angina episodes, as these act as adenosine receptor blockers; adenosine being a major mediator of cardiac ischaemic pain.

New anti-ischaemic drugs such as ranolazine or ivabradine have been reported to be of help in MVA. Ranolazine is a relatively new drug that exerts its anti-ischemic effects by inhibiting the inward late sodium current in cardiomyocytes; this results in a reduction of intracellular calcium inflow during ischemia, with improvement of myocardial relaxation and ventricular diastolic function. Data suggest that ranolazine may improve endothelial function [72]. In clinical trials, ranolazine improved symptoms and exercise performance in angina patients with obstructive coronary artery disease [73]. Lanza et al. randomized 45 patients with MVA with symptoms not satisfactorily controlled by standard medical therapy to receive ranolazine, ivabradine, or placebo for 4 weeks. Ranolazine, but not placebo, significantly improved angina symptoms and quality of life, as well as exercise stress test results. The improvement observed in this study was significantly better for ranolazine compared with ivabradine 5 mg bid [74]. The results of this study are in agreement with those of a crossover trial of 20 women with chest pain and normal coronary arteries, in whom angina symptoms were improved by ranolazine in the subgroup showing a reduced myocardial perfusion reserve [75].

Recently, Bairey Merz et al. [76] reported the results of a double-blind, placebo-controlled, crossover trial of ranolazine in patients with chest pain symptoms thought to be caused by myocardial ischaemia, absence of obstructive coronary artery disease at angiography (no stenosis >50 % in epicardial coronary arteries), and evidence of CMD, as suggested by at least one of the following findings: (i) invasive coronary flow reserve (CFR) to adenosine <2.5; (ii) no dilatation (≤ 0 % change) in response to acetylcholine (Ach); and (iii) myocardial perfusion reserve index (MPRI) <2.0 on pharmacological cardiac magnetic resonance imaging (CMRI) stress test.

Ranolazine (500 mg twice a day, possibly increased to 1 g twice a day) or placebo were given in random sequence for 2 weeks each. Clinical status was carefully and extensively evaluated, using standardised questionnaires and an angina diary. Gadolinium CMRI was performed to assess myocardial perfusion at rest and during a pharmacological (adenosine or regadenoson) stress test and cold pressor test. No differences in the primary endpoints were found between ranolazine and placebo, including Seattle angina questionnaire (SAQ) scores and angina episodes or nitroglycerin use, although the QoL depression score significantly improved with ranolazine but not with placebo. No significant effects were observed, with either ranolazione or placebo, on stress CMRI results. Interestingly, among 78 subjects with available invasive adenosine CFR data, those with baseline CFR <2.5 had significantly higher midventricular stress MPRI improvement as compared with those with CFR 2.5–3.0 and >3.0. This improvement was paralleled by an improvement of SAQ angina frequency and global SAQ-7 score. Furthermore, significant, albeit modest, correlations were found between changes in global or subendocardial MPRI and changes in some SAQ and QoL scores with ranolazine vs. placebo, even after adjustment for potential confounders.

The data demonstrate that ranolazine does not improve symptoms or objective signs of myocardial ischaemia in an unselected population of patients with MVA. A novel observation is that in this patient population symptomatic improvement with ranolazine correlated with changes in MPRI, thus giving strong support to the notion that angina was caused by CMD. A major limitation of the study is the inclusion of a non-selected and heterogeneous population of patients with a diagnosis of MVA. Thus, the benefit of ranolazine in patients with low CFR, as shown by subgroup post-hoc analyses, was probably diluted by the lack of efficacy in the remaining patients, as suggested by Crea et al. in a recent editorial article [77].

Ivabradine is also a relatively new anti-ischemic drug, which has been shown to improve angina symptoms in several clinical trials of patients with obstructive CAD [78]. Ivabradine is a selective heart rate reducing agent that acts by reducing pacemaker activity of the sinus node through inhibition of the If current, thus resulting in a reduced myocardial oxygen consumption, both at rest and during exercise. In a study by Lanza et al. [74], ivabradine significantly improved angina status in MVA patients compared with placebo, although its effects were less marked than those found with ranolazine.

Management of Pain Perception Abnormalities in MVA

While CMD can be detected in most patients with chest pain and signs of myocardial ischaemia, despite no obstructive coronary artery disease at angiography, a subset of patients has consistently been found to have enhanced pain perception. These subjects have an exaggerated response to stimuli which do not elicit severe pain in patients with coronary artery disease [79]. These stimuli include intracardiac saline or contrast medium injection, catheter manipulation within the heart chambers, and electrical ventricular stimulation [80]. This increased cardiac pain sensitivity may contribute to symptom severity, and the development of chest pain even in the presence of mild microvascular ischaemia [3].

These diverse causes of angina in MVA patients may have a different relevance in different patients, and it may be the reason why standard pharmacological anti-ischaemic treatment is often disappointing in patients with chest pain and normal coronary arteries. Approximately 25 % of patients, have recurrent angina with impaired quality of life (QoL), associated with frequent re-hospitalization and repeat non-invasive investigation and coronary angiography, in spite of multiple drug therapy [81].

Pharmacological Treatment of Pain in MVA

Drugs that inhibit transmission and processing of visceral pain might be helpful in patients with MVA who are resistant to anti-ischemic treatment, particularly when an enhanced painful perception of cardiac stimuli is present, as described above [80, 82]. The centrally acting analgesic imipramine was assessed in two controlled trials. In a study of patients with chest pain and normal coronary arteries, the drug reduced chest pain attacks by 52 ± 25 % over a period of 3 weeks [83], whereas no significant effects were observed with placebo or clonidine. This effect of imipramine on angina episodes was confirmed in a second trial including typical MVA patients [84]; however, imipramine did not improve quality of life, probably due to a significant occurrence of side effects. Thus, although imipramine seems useful to prevent episodes of chest pain, the frequent occurrence of side effects can significantly limit its use.

Non-pharmacological Treatment

In some cases, chest pain episodes may persist despite pharmacological treatment. In these cases of 'refractory MVA', alternative non-pharmacological approaches have been suggested. Among these, spinal cord stimulation (SCS) and Enhanced External Counterpulsation (EECP) are the most common. SCS involves the electrical stimulation of the dorsal horns of the spinal cord at C7-T1 level by a multipolar electrode catheter implanted in the epidural space. A programmable pulse generator, usually implanted in a subcutaneous abdominal or gluteal pocket, allows the delivery of electrical pulses. SCS seems to exert its anti-angina effects through both direct modulation of cardiac pain transmission and the improvement of myocardial ischemia. The latter is probably achieved through modulatory effects of sympathetic nerve activity [85]. In MVA patients SCS has been shown to improve both ischaemic and angina thresholds, as well as exercise tolerance and the development of spontaneous ischemic episodes [86–88]. A reduction in nitrate consumption, and improved quality of life have been also reported to occur in a controlled study [89]. Accordingly, SCS should be considered in MVA patients refractory to various forms of medical therapy.

EECP consists of a sequential beat-by-beat distal to proximal inflation (in diastole) and deflation (in systole) of three pneumatic cuffs applied to the patient's legs. This results in increased diastolic coronary perfusion pressure, which seems to improve perfusion and coronary endothelial function [90]. In a study of 30 patients with refractory MVA, EECP has been shown to improve angina and myocardial ischemia [91]. However, larger controlled studies are needed to better define the role of EECP in MVA. The treatment is poorly tolerated by some patients and it can also be associated with other unwanted side effects such as headache and dyspnoea [92].

Other Supportive Measures

Exercise rehabilitation programs have been shown to improve symptoms in MVA patients [93], and should therefore be recommended to patients with symptoms refractory to pharmacological treatment. Psychologic interventions can also be helpful in the management of refractory MVA [94]. Various types of psychological intervention assessed in small studies have been shown to reduce psychologic morbidity and improve quality of life [95].

References

1. Patel MR, Peterson ED, Dai D, Brennan JM, Redberg RF, Anderson HV, Brindis RG, Douglas PS. Low diagnostic yield of elective coronary angiography. N Engl J Med. 2010;362:886–95.
2. Douglas PS, Patel MR, Bailey SR, Dai D, Kaltenbach L, Brindis RG, Messenger J, Peterson ED. Hospital variability in the rate of finding obstructive coronary artery disease at elective, diagnostic coronary angiography. J Am Coll Cardiol. 2011;58:801–9.
3. Kaski JC. Pathophysiology and management of patients with chest pain and normal coronary arteriograms (cardiac syndrome X). Circulation. 2004;109:568–72.
4. Maseri A, Crea F, Kaski JC, Crake T. Mechanisms of angina pectoris in syndrome X. J Am Coll Cardiol. 1991;17:499–506.
5. Cannon RO, Camici PG, Epstein SE. Pathophysiological dilemma of syndrome X. Circulation. 1992;85:883–92.
6. Cannon RO, Epstein SE. 'Microvascular angina' as a cause of chest pain with angiographically normal coronary arteries. Am J Cardiol. 1988;61:1338–43.
7. Lanza GA, Crea F. Primary coronary microvascular dysfunction: clinical presentation, pathophysiology, and management. Circulation. 2010;121:2317–25.

8. Herrmann J, Kaski JC, Lerman A. Coronary microvascular dysfunction in the clinical setting: from mystery to reality. Eur Heart J. 2012;33:2771–83.

9. Crea F, Camici PG, Bairey Merz CN. Coronary microvascular dysfunction: an update. Eur Heart J. 2014;35:1101–11.

10. Radico F, Cicchitti V, Zimarino M, De Caterina R. Angina pectoris and myocardial ischemia in the absence of obstructive coronary artery disease: practical considerations for diagnostic tests. JACC Cardiovasc Interv. 2014;7:453–63.

11. Camici PG, Crea F. Coronary microvascular dysfunction. N Engl J Med. 2007;356:830–40.

12. Panting JR, Gatehouse PD, Yang G-Z, Grothues F, Firmin DN, Collins P, Pennell DJ. Abnormal subendocardial perfusion in cardiac syndrome X detected by cardiovascular magnetic resonance imaging. N Engl J Med. 2002;346:1948–53.

13. Kaski JC, Rosano GM, Collins P, Nihoyannopoulos P, Maseri A, Poole-Wilson PA. Cardiac syndrome X: clinical characteristics and left ventricular function. Long-term follow-up study. J Am Coll Cardiol. 1995;25:807–14.

14. Lanza GA, Manzoli A, Bia E, Crea F, Maseri A. Acute effects of nitrates on exercise testing in patients with syndrome X. Clinical and pathophysiological implications. Circulation. 1994;90:2695–700.

15. Ong P, Athanasiadis A, Borgulya G, Mahrholdt H, Kaski JC, Sechtem U. High prevalence of a pathological response to acetylcholine testing in patients with stable angina pectoris and unobstructed coronary arteries. The ACOVA Study (Abnormal COronary VAsomotion in patients with stable angina and unobstructed coronary arteries. J Am Coll Cardiol. 2012;59:655–62.

16. Kanatsuka H, Eastham CL, Marcus ML, Lamping KG. Effects of nitroglycerin on the coronary microcirculation in normal and ischemic myocardium. J Cardiovasc Pharmacol. 1992;19:755–63.

17. Infusino F, Lanza GA, Sestito A, Sgueglia GA, Crea F, Maseri A. Combination of variant and microvascular angina. Clin Cardiol. 2009;32:E40–5.

18. Kaski JC, Aldama G, Cosín-Sales J. Cardiac syndrome X. Diagnosis, pathogenesis and management. Am J Cardiovasc Drugs. 2004;4:179–94.

19. Nihoyannopoulos P, Kaski JC, Crake T, Maseri A. Absence of myocardial dysfunction during stress in patients with syndrome X. J Am Coll Cardiol. 1991;18:1463–70.

20. Panza JA, Laurienzo JM, Curiel RV, Unger EF, Quyyumi AA, Dilsizian V, Cannon RO. Investigation of the mechanism of chest pain in patients with angiographically normal coronary arteries using transesophageal dobutamine stress echocardiography. J Am Coll Cardiol. 1997;29:293–301.
21. Wu KC, Zerhouni EA, Judd RM, Lugo-Olivieri CH, Barouch LA, Schulman SP, Blumenthal RS, Lima JA. Prognostic significance of microvascular obstruction by magnetic resonance imaging in patients with acute myocardial infarction. Circulation. 1998;97:765–72.
22. Leung DY, Leung M. Non-invasive/invasive imaging: significance and assessment of coronary microvascular dysfunction. Heart. 2011;97:587–95.
23. Cassar A, Chareonthaitawee P, Rihal CS, Prasad A, Lennon RJ, Lerman LO, Lerman A. Lack of correlation between noninvasive stress tests and invasive coronary vasomotor dysfunction in patients with nonobstructive coronary artery disease. Circ Cardiovasc Interv. 2009;2:237–44.
24. Gibson CM, Cannon CP, Daley WL, Dodge JT, Alexander B, Marble SJ, McCabe CH, Raymond L, Fortin T, Poole WK, Braunwald E. TIMI frame count: a quantitative method of assessing coronary artery flow. Circulation. 1996;93:879–88.
25. Pijls NHJ, De Bruyne B, Smith L, Aarnoudse W, Barbato E, Bartunek J, Bech GJW, Van De Vosse F. Coronary thermodilution to assess flow reserve: validation in humans. Circulation. 2002;105:2482–6.
26. Fearon WF, Balsam LB, Farouque HMO, Caffarelli AD, Robbins RC, Fitzgerald PJ, Yock PG, Yeung AC. Novel index for invasively assessing the coronary microcirculation. Circulation. 2003;107:3129–32.
27. Melikian N, Kearney MT, Thomas MR, De Bruyne B, Shah AM, MacCarthy PA. A simple thermodilution technique to assess coronary endothelium-dependent microvascular function in humans: validation and comparison with coronary flow reserve. Eur Heart J. 2007;28:2188–94.
28. Yong ASC, Ho M, Shah MG, Ng MKC, Fearon WF. Coronary microcirculatory resistance is independent of epicardial stenosis. Circ Cardiovasc Interv. 2012;5:103–8, S1–2.
29. Herrmann J, Lerman A. The endothelium: dysfunction and beyond. J Nucl Cardiol. 2001;8:197–206.
30. Newby DE. Intracoronary infusions and the assessment of coronary blood flow in clinical studies. Heart. 2000;84:118–20.

31. Papanicolaou MN, Califf RM, Hlatky MA, McKinnis RA, Harrell FE, Mark DB, McCants B, Rosati RA, Lee KL, Pryor DB. Prognostic implications of angiographically normal and insignificantly narrowed coronary arteries. Am J Cardiol. 1986;58:1181–7.

32. Lichtlen PR, Bargheer K, Wenzlaff P. Long-term prognosis of patients with anginalike chest pain and normal coronary angiographic findings. J Am Coll Cardiol. 1995;25:1013–8.

33. Kemp HG, Kronmal RA, Vlietstra RE, Frye RL. Seven year survival of patients with normal or near normal coronary arteriograms: a CASS registry study. J Am Coll Cardiol. 1986;7:479–83.

34. Proudfit WL, Bruschke VG, Sones FM. Clinical course of patients with normal or slightly or moderately abnormal coronary arteriograms: 10-year follow-up of 521 patients. Circulation. 1980;62:712–7.

35. Pepine CJ, Anderson RD, Sharaf BL, Reis SE, Smith KM, Handberg EM, Johnson BD, Sopko G, Bairey Merz CN. Coronary microvascular reactivity to adenosine predicts adverse outcome in women evaluated for suspected ischemia results from the National Heart, Lung and Blood Institute WISE (Women's Ischemia Syndrome Evaluation) study. J Am Coll Cardiol. 2010;55:2825–32.

36. Pepine CJ, Kerensky RA, National Heart, Lung and Blood Institute. Abnormal coronary vasomotion as a prognostic indicator of cardiovascular events in women: results from the National Heart, Lung, and Blood Institute-Sponsored Women's Ischemia Syndrome Evaluation (WISE). Circulation. 2004;109:722–5.

37. Herzog BA, Husmann L, Valenta I, Gaemperli O, Siegrist PT, Tay FM, Burkhard N, Wyss CA, Kaufmann PA. Long-term prognostic value of 13N-ammonia myocardial perfusion positron emission tomography added value of coronary flow reserve. J Am Coll Cardiol. 2009;54:150–6.

38. Schindler TH, Nitzsche EU, Schelbert HR, Olschewski M, Sayre J, Mix M, Brink I, Zhang X-L, Kreissl M, Magosaki N, Just H, Solzbach U. Positron emission tomography-measured abnormal responses of myocardial blood flow to sympathetic stimulation are associated with the risk of developing cardiovascular events. J Am Coll Cardiol. 2005;45:1505–12.

39. Murthy VL, Naya M, Taqueti VR, Foster CR, Gaber M, Hainer J, Dorbala S, Blankstein R, Rimoldi O, Camici PG, Di Carli MF. Effects of sex on coronary microvascular dysfunction and cardiac outcomes. Circulation. 2014;129:2518–27.

40. Jespersen L, Hvelplund A, Abildstrøm SZ, Pedersen F, Galatius S, Madsen JK, Jørgensen E, Kelbæk H, Prescott E. Stable angina pectoris with no obstructive coronary artery disease is associated with increased risks of major adverse cardiovascular events. Eur Heart J. 2012;33:734–44.
41. Lanza GA, Parrinello R, Figliozzi S. Management of microvascular angina pectoris. Am J Cardiovasc Drugs. 2014;14:31–40.
42. Cannon RO, Watson RM, Rosing DR, Epstein SE. Efficacy of calcium channel blocker therapy for angina pectoris resulting from small-vessel coronary artery disease and abnormal vasodilator reserve. Am J Cardiol. 1985;56:242–6.
43. Ozçelik F, Altun A, Ozbay G. Antianginal and anti-ischemic effects of nisoldipine and ramipril in patients with syndrome X. Clin Cardiol. 1999;22:361–5.
44. Li L, Gu Y, Liu T, Bai Y, Hou L, Cheng Z, Hu L, Gao B. A randomized, single-center double-blinded trial on the effects of diltiazem sustained-release capsules in patients with coronary slow flow phenomenon at 6-month follow-up. PLoS One. 2012;7:e38851.
45. Lanza GA, Colonna G, Pasceri V, Maseri A. Atenolol versus amlodipine versus isosorbide-5-mononitrate on anginal symptoms in syndrome X. Am J Cardiol. 1999;84:854–6, A8.
46. Romeo F, Gaspardone A, Ciavolella M, Gioffrè P, Reale A. Verapamil versus acebutolol for syndrome X. Am J Cardiol. 1988;62:312–3.
47. Ferrini D, Bugiardini R, Galvani M, Gridelli C, Tollemeto D, Puddu P, Lenzi S. Opposing effects of propranolol and diltiazem on the angina threshold during an exercise test in patients with syndrome X. G Ital Cardiol. 1986;16:224–31.
48. Montorsi P, Cozzi S, Loaldi A, Fabbiocchi F, Polese A, De Cesare N, Guazzi MD. Acute coronary vasomotor effects of nifedipine and therapeutic correlates in syndrome X. Am J Cardiol. 1990;66:302–7.
49. Hill JA, Feldman RL, Pepine CJ, Conti CR. Randomized double-blind comparison of nifedipine and isosorbide dinitrate in patients with coronary arterial spasm. Am J Cardiol. 1982;49:431–8.
50. Lablanche JM, Bauters C, Leroy F, Bertrand ME. Prevention of coronary spasm by nicorandil: comparison with nifedipine. J Cardiovasc Pharmacol. 1992;20 Suppl 3:S82–5.
51. Takahashi J, Nihei T, Takagi Y, Miyata S, Odaka Y, Tsunoda R, Seki A, Sumiyoshi T, Matsui M, Goto T, Tanabe Y, Sueda S, Momomura S, Yasuda S, Ogawa H, Shimokawa H, Japanese

Coronary Spasm Association. Prognostic impact of chronic nitrate therapy in patients with vasospastic angina: multicentre registry study of the Japanese coronary spasm association. Eur Heart J. 2015;36:228–37.

52. Russo G, Di Franco A, Lamendola P, Tarzia P, Nerla R, Stazi A, Villano A, Sestito A, Lanza GA, Crea F. Lack of effect of nitrates on exercise stress test results in patients with microvascular angina. Cardiovasc Drugs Ther. 2013;27:229–34.

53. Yamabe H, Namura H, Yano T, Fujita H, Kim S, Iwahashi M, Maeda K, Yokoyama M. Effect of nicorandil on abnormal coronary flow reserve assessed by exercise 201Tl scintigraphy in patients with angina pectoris and nearly normal coronary arteriograms. Cardiovasc Drugs Ther. 1995;9:755–61.

54. Kaski JC, Valenzuela Garcia LF. Therapeutic options for the management of patients with cardiac syndrome X. Eur Heart J. 2001;22:283–93.

55. Sadamatsu K, Tashiro H, Yoshida K, Shikada T, Iwamoto K, Morishige K, Yoshidomi Y, Tokunou T, Tanaka H. Acute effects of isosorbide dinitrate and nicorandil on the coronary slow flow phenomenon. Am J Cardiovasc Drugs. 2010;10:203–8.

56. Chen JW, Lee WL, Hsu NW, Lin SJ, Ting CT, Wang SP, Chang MS. Effects of short-term treatment of nicorandil on exercise-induced myocardial ischemia and abnormal cardiac autonomic activity in microvascular angina. Am J Cardiol. 1997;80:32–8.

57. Pizzi C, Manfrini O, Fontana F, Bugiardini R. Angiotensin-converting enzyme inhibitors and 3-hydroxy-3-methylglutaryl coenzyme A reductase in cardiac Syndrome X: role of superoxide dismutase activity. Circulation. 2004;109:53–8.

58. Pauly DF, Johnson BD, Anderson RD, Handberg EM, Smith KM, Cooper-DeHoff RM, Sopko G, Sharaf BM, Kelsey SF, Merz CNB, Pepine CJ. In women with symptoms of cardiac ischemia, nonobstructive coronary arteries, and microvascular dysfunction, angiotensin-converting enzyme inhibition is associated with improved microvascular function: a double-blind randomized study from the National Hea. Am Heart J. 2011;162:678–84.

59. Kaski JC, Rosano G, Gavrielides S, Chen L. Effects of angiotensin-converting enzyme inhibition on exercise-induced angina and ST segment depression in patients with microvascular angina. J Am Coll Cardiol. 1994;23:652–7.

60. Nalbantgil I, Onder R, Altintig A, Nalbantgil S, Kiliçcioglu B, Boydak B, Yilmaz H. Therapeutic benefits of cilazapril in patients with syndrome X. Cardiology. 1998;89:130–3.

61. Chen J-W, Hsu N-W, Wu T-C, Lin S-J, Chang M-S. Long-term angiotensin-converting enzyme inhibition reduces plasma asymmetric dimethylarginine and improves endothelial nitric oxide bioavailability and coronary microvascular function in patients with syndrome X. Am J Cardiol. 2002;90:974–82.

62. Camici PG, Marraccini P, Gistri R, Salvadori PA, Sorace O, L'Abbate A. Adrenergically mediated coronary vasoconstriction in patients with syndrome X. Cardiovasc Drugs Ther. 1994;8:221–6.

63. Rosen SD, Lorenzoni R, Kaski JC, Foale RA, Camici PG. Effect of alpha1-adrenoceptor blockade on coronary vasodilator reserve in cardiac syndrome X. J Cardiovasc Pharmacol. 1999;34:554–60.

64. Galassi AR, Kaski JC, Pupita G, Vejar M, Crea F, Maseri A. Lack of evidence for alpha-adrenergic receptor-mediated mechanisms in the genesis of ischemia in syndrome X. Am J Cardiol. 1989;64:264–9.

65. Fábián E, Varga A, Picano E, Vajo Z, Rónaszéki A, Csanády M. Effect of simvastatin on endothelial function in cardiac syndrome X patients. Am J Cardiol. 2004;94:652–5.

66. Albertsson PA, Emanuelsson H, Milsom I. Beneficial effect of treatment with transdermal estradiol-17-beta on exercise-induced angina and ST segment depression in syndrome X. Int J Cardiol. 1996;54:13–20.

67. Lanza GA, Giordano A, Pristipino C, Calcagni ML, Meduri G, Trani C, Franceschini R, Crea F, Troncone L, Maseri A. Abnormal cardiac adrenergic nerve function in patients with syndrome X detected by [123I]metaiodobenzylguanidine myocardial scintigraphy. Circulation. 1997;96:821–6.

68. Collins P. Role of endothelial dysfunction and oestrogens in syndrome X. Coron Artery Dis. 1992;3:593–8.

69. Rosano GM, Peters NS, Lefroy D, Lindsay DC, Sarrel PM, Collins P, Poole-Wilson PA. 17-beta-Estradiol therapy lessens angina in postmenopausal women with syndrome X. J Am Coll Cardiol. 1996;28:1500–5.

70. Jhund PS, Dawson N, Davie AP, Sattar N, Norrie J, O'Kane KP, McMurray JJ. Attenuation of endothelin-1 induced vasoconstriction by 17beta estradiol is not sustained during long-term therapy in postmenopausal women with coronary heart disease. J Am Coll Cardiol. 2001;37:1367–73.

71. Anderson GL, Limacher M, Assaf AR, Bassford T, Beresford SAA, Black H, Bonds D, Brunner R, Brzyski R, Caan B,

Chlebowski R, Curb D, Gass M, Hays J, Heiss G, Hendrix S, Howard BV, Hsia J, Hubbell A, Jackson R, Johnson KC, Judd H, Kotchen JM, Kuller L, LaCroix AZ, Lane D, Langer RD, Lasser N, Lewis CE, Manson J, et al. Effects of conjugated equine estrogen in postmenopausal women with hysterectomy: the Women's Health Initiative randomized controlled trial. JAMA. 2004;291:1701–12.

72. Lamendola P, Nerla R, Pitocco D, Villano A, Scavone G, Stazi A, Russo G, Di Franco A, Sestito A, Ghirlanda G, Lanza GA, Crea F. Effect of ranolazine on arterial endothelial function in patients with type 2 diabetes mellitus. Atherosclerosis. 2013;226:157–60.

73. Keating GM. Ranolazine: a review of its use in chronic stable angina pectoris. Drugs. 2008;68:2483–503.

74. Villano A, Di Franco A, Nerla R, Sestito A, Tarzia P, Lamendola P, Di Monaco A, Sarullo FM, Lanza GA, Crea F. Effects of ivabradine and ranolazine in patients with microvascular angina pectoris. Am J Cardiol. 2013;112:8–13.

75. Mehta PK, Goykhman P, Thomson LEJ, Shufelt C, Wei J, Yang Y, Gill E, Minissian M, Shaw LJ, Slomka PJ, Slivka M, Berman DS, Bairey Merz CN. Ranolazine improves angina in women with evidence of myocardial ischemia but no obstructive coronary artery disease. JACC Cardiovasc Imaging. 2011;4:514–22.

76. Bairey Merz CN, Handberg EM, Shufelt CL, Mehta PK, Minissian MB, Wei J, Thomson LEJ, Berman DS, Shaw LJ, Petersen JW, Brown GH, Anderson RD, Shuster JJ, Cook-Wiens G, Rogatko A, Pepine CJ. A randomized, placebo-controlled trial of late Na current inhibition (ranolazine) in coronary microvascular dysfunction (CMD): impact on angina and myocardial perfusion reserve. Eur Heart J. 2016;37(19):1504–13.

77. Crea F, Lanza GA. Treatment of microvascular angina: the need for precision medicine. Eur Heart J. 2016. doi:10.1093/eurheartj/ehw021.

78. Borer JS, Fox K, Jaillon P, Lerebours G, Ivabradine Investigators Group. Antianginal and antiischemic effects of ivabradine, an I(f) inhibitor, in stable angina: a randomized, double-blind, multi-centered, placebo-controlled trial. Circulation. 2003;107:817–23.

79. Benjamin SB. Microvascular angina and the sensitive heart: historical perspective. Am J Med. 1992;92:52S–5.

80. Pasceri V, Lanza GA, Buffon A, Montenero AS, Crea F, Maseri A. Role of abnormal pain sensitivity and behavioral factors in determining chest pain in syndrome X. J Am Coll Cardiol. 1998;31:62–6.

81. Lamendola P, Lanza GA, Spinelli A, Sgueglia GA, Di Monaco A, Barone L, Sestito A, Crea F. Long-term prognosis of patients with cardiac syndrome X. Int J Cardiol. 2010;140:197–9.
82. Cannon RO, Quyyumi AA, Schenke WH, Fananapazir L, Tucker EE, Gaughan AM, Gracely RH, Cattau EL, Epstein SE. Abnormal cardiac sensitivity in patients with chest pain and normal coronary arteries. J Am Coll Cardiol. 1990;16:1359–66.
83. Cannon RO, Quyyumi AA, Mincemoyer R, Stine AM, Gracely RH, Smith WB, Geraci MF, Black BC, Uhde TW, Waclawiw MA. Imipramine in patients with chest pain despite normal coronary angiograms. N Engl J Med. 1994;330:1411–7.
84. Cox ID, Hann CM, Kaski JC. Low dose imipramine improves chest pain but not quality of life in patients with angina and normal coronary angiograms. Eur Heart J. 1998;19:250–4.
85. Norrsell H, Eliasson T, Mannheimer C, Augustinsson LE, Bergh CH, Andersson B, Waagstein F, Friberg P. Effects of pacing-induced myocardial stress and spinal cord stimulation on whole body and cardiac norepinephrine spillover. Eur Heart J. 1997;18:1890–6.
86. Eliasson T, Albertsson P, Hårdhammar P, Emanuelsson H, Augustinsson LE, Mannheimer C. Spinal cord stimulation in angina pectoris with normal coronary arteriograms. Coron Artery Dis. 1993;4:819–27.
87. Lanza GA, Sestito A, Sandric S, Cioni B, Tamburrini G, Barollo A, Crea F, De Seta F, Meglio M, Bellocci F, Maseri A. Spinal cord stimulation in patients with refractory anginal pain and normal coronary arteries. Ital Heart J. 2001;2:25–30.
88. Lanza GA, Sestito A, Sgueglia GA, Infusino F, Papacci F, Visocchi M, Ierardi C, Meglio M, Bellocci F, Crea F. Effect of spinal cord stimulation on spontaneous and stress-induced angina and 'ischemia-like' ST-segment depression in patients with cardiac syndrome X. Eur Heart J. 2005;26:983–9.
89. Sgueglia GA, Sestito A, Spinelli A, Cioni B, Infusino F, Papacci F, Bellocci F, Meglio M, Crea F, Lanza GA. Long-term follow-up of patients with cardiac syndrome X treated by spinal cord stimulation. Heart. 2007;93:591–7.
90. Kitsou V, Xanthos T, Roberts R, Karlis GM, Padadimitriou L. Enhanced external counterpulsation: mechanisms of action and clinical applications. Acta Cardiol. 2010;65:239–47.
91. Kronhaus KD, Lawson WE. Enhanced external counterpulsation is an effective treatment for Syndrome X. Int J Cardiol. 2009;135:256–7.

92. Lanza GA. Alternative treatments for angina. Heart. 2007;93:544–6.
93. Asbury EA, Slattery C, Grant A, Evans L, Barbir M, Collins P. Cardiac rehabilitation for the treatment of women with chest pain and normal coronary arteries. Menopause. 2008;15:454–60.
94. Bass C, Wade C. Chest pain with normal coronary arteries: a comparative study of psychiatric and social morbidity. Psychol Med. 1984;14:51–61.
95. Potts SG, Lewin R, Fox KA, Johnstone EC. Group psychological treatment for chest pain with normal coronary arteries. QJM. 1999;92:81–6.

Chapter 5
Angina in Women

Abstract   Ischemic heart disease has been shown to equally affect men and women, albeit the condition becomes manifest approximately a decade later in women compared with men. Among the elderly, the absolute number of women affected by angina pectoris is greater than that in men. Moreover, mortality rates associated with cerebrovascular and cardiovascular disease are higher in women compared with men, and recent observations indicate that while mortality appears to be declining in men this is not the case among women. Cardiovascular disease is now recognized as the leading cause of death for women in developed countries worldwide and is more common than death from cancer, HIV, malaria and tuberculosis combined. The prevalence of angina pectoris in the absence of obstructive CAD is higher in women compared with men. Hypertension is more prevalent in elderly women than in men and this has been suggested to represent an explanation for the higher prevalence of stroke and heart failure with preserved ejection fraction in women compared with male patients. Similarly, studies have reported that women with type 2 diabetes have a higher risk of cardiovascular mortality than women with no diabetes and diabetic men. The differences in clinical outcome between men and women have been attributed to a greater prevalence of risk factors, inflammation, diffuse coronary atherosclerosis and small vessel disease, in diabetic women than in diabetic men. Differences in diagnostic strategies and treatment

J.C. Kaski, *Essentials in Stable Angina Pectoris*,
DOI 10.1007/978-3-319-41180-4_5,
© Springer International Publishing Switzerland 2016

disparities, favouring men, may represent another important factor. These issues will be discussed in this chapter.

Introduction

In recent years it has become apparent that ischemic heart disease (IHD) equally affects men and women [1–3], albeit the condition becomes manifest approximately a decade later in the latter [4, 5]. Among the elderly, the absolute number of females with angina pectoris is greater than that of males [4]. Moreover, mortality rates associated with cerebrovascular and cardiovascular disease are higher in women compared with men [2, 3], and recent observations indicate that while mortality appears to be declining in men this is not the case among women [4]. The important topic of angina in women has been recently reviewed by F Crea et al. [6] and by K. Schenck-Gustafsson [7].

Epidemiology

Prevalence

For several years it has been known that stable angina is the most common initial symptomatic presentation of IHD among women [8]. Cardiovascular disease is now recognized as the leading cause of death for women in developed countries worldwide and is more common than death from cancer, HIV, malaria and tuberculosis combined [9]. It is estimated that 50 % of deaths among women are associated with heart disease or stroke, while 1 in 25 die of breast cancer [10, 11]. This is contrary to perception among patients and physicians that women are not so dramatically affected by IHD [8, 12].

As recently reported by K. Schenck-Gustafsson [7], an international study involving 31 countries showed a higher prevalence of angina in women transnationally, with estimates of 6.7 % in women versus 5.6 % in men [10]. In a large epidemiological study in a Finnish population, including

56,441 women and 34,885 men, the prevalence of angina pectoris was similar in men and women. Moreover, the age-standardized annual incidence of all cases of angina, per 100 population, was 2.03 in men and 1.89 in women, with a sex ratio of 1.07 (95 % CI 1.06–1.09). Stable angina in women was associated with increased coronary mortality compared with women in the general population. Clinical outcomes were similar in men and women [11].

The prevalence of angina pectoris in the absence of obstructive CAD is higher in women compared with men. The Coronary Artery Surgery Study (CASS) registry involving approximately 25,000 patients undergoing coronary angiography for angina, showed no obstructive CAD in 39 % of women compared with 11 % of men [13]. In the Women's Ischemic Syndrome Evaluation (WISE) study, 62 % of women referred for angiography had no obstructive CAD [14], and among 375,886 patients undergoing angiography for assessment of stable angina (The American College of Cardiology-National Cardiovascular Data Registry – NCDR) the prevalence of angina with no obstructive CAD was significantly higher in women (51 %) than in men (32 %) [12]. Data from Europe have shown similar results [15].

Regarding acute coronary artery disease, recent surveys showed an increased prevalence of myocardial infarction in younger women, i.e. 35–54 years of age, and a decline among men of a similar age [16]. The reasons for these trends, as suggested by Crea et al. [6], are likely to by multiple, including increasing unhealthy lifestyle changes among women, management biases and increased awareness of the existence of the disease among women [17].

Women-specific recommendations for the management and prevention of cardiovascular disease have been issued by American and European organisations [2, 18].

Of interest, studies in both acute coronary syndrome patients and chronic stable angina have shown that women tend to have a higher prevalence of non-obstructive coronary artery disease compared with men, i.e. 20 % and 10 %, respectively [19].

Financial Burden of Angina Pectoris in Women

Data from the American Heart Association indicate that over nine million people in the United States suffer from angina pectoris, which significantly affects quality of life and working practice, and represents a serious financial burden to health services [20].

Shaw et al. indicated that for women with angina, the burden of symptoms and ongoing treatment for risk factors results in a heavy economic burden. In the WISE registry, Shaw and colleagues reported 5-year costs for cardiovascular disease ranging from 32,000 to 53,000 US dollars for women with non-obstructive to multi-vessel CAD [14]. Projections from these results, according to Shaw et al. [14], indicate that even women with mild CAD or non-obstructive CAD would spend nearly 750,000 US dollars during their lifetime. As reviewed by Johnston et al. the high cost of care was due to the presence and persistence of ongoing anginal symptoms [15]. In fact, the costs of anti-anginal drug therapy was higher for women with non-obstructive CAD as compared to those with obstructive CAD ($p = 0.004$). These results support the concept that ongoing symptoms drive the costs of care. In a related report, persistent chest pain was found to be frequent in women despite anti-anginal treatment [21]. It was calculated that nearly 50% of the women presenting for assessment of a de novo chest pain will continue to have angina symptoms at 5 years of follow-up [14].

These data taken together clearly indicate that high costs of care are heavily influenced by chest pain symptoms and the need for repeated diagnostic tests.

Cardiovascular Risk Factors in Women

Hypertension is more prevalent in elderly women than in men and this has been suggested to represent an explanation for the higher prevalence of stroke and heart failure with preserved ejection fraction in women compared with male patients [22]. Similarly, studies have reported that women with type 2 diabetes have a higher risk of cardiovascular mortality than women with no diabetes and diabetic males [23–25].

As reviewed by Crea et al. [6], the differences in clinical outcome between men and women have been attributed to a greater prevalence of risk factors, inflammation, diffuse coronary atherosclerosis and small vessel disease, in diabetic women than in diabetic men [23–25]. Differences in diagnostic strategies and treatment disparities, favouring men, may represent another important factor [6].

According to Andreotti and Marchese [4], European and American risk estimation tools for individual cardiovascular risk suggest that for any given risk factor or their combination, the likelihood of future adverse events is generally lower among apparently healthy women than among age-matched men. However, if the burden of risk factors would be higher among women compared with men this could explain some of the findings depicted above. Andreotti suggests that the prevalence of all risk factors except smoking is typically greater among female than among age-matched male patients, "given that IHD 'selects' women with a cluster of risk factors" [4]. The Study Of Risk Factors For First Myocardial Infarction in 52 Countries And Over 27,000 Subjects (INTERHEART) showed increased odds ratios for myocardial infarction among female than male patients, with a higher risk factor burden regarding hypertension, diabetes, exercise, and alcohol, among others [26]. As suggested by K. Schenck-Gustafsson [7], analysis of risk factors in women should include "not only the traditional risk factors such as dyslipidaemia, hypertension, smoking, diabetes mellitus, stress, obesity, physical inactivity, unhealthy diet and alcohol intake" but also women specific factors. Among these, premature menopause, polycystic ovary syndrome, gestational diabetes, preeclampsia and eclampsia have to be considered. In women with microvascular angina and non-obstructive coronary artery disease or in the absence of obstructive CAD, oestrogen deficiency and insulin resistance are likely to play a predisposing role.

Differences in Clinical Presentation and Diagnosis

Stable angina pectoris is the most common form of presentation of IHD disease in both men and women. With the excep-
tion of the ARIC study, [27] most studies indicate a higher
prevalence and incidence of angina pectoris in men than in
women [4, 5, 28, 29]. Compared with men, women with angina
pectoris present at an older age, and are more frequently
hypertensive [30, 31], but have a lower prevalence of smoking
and previous infarction. Angina equivalents and associated
symptoms in women with angina, as reported by Shaw et al.
[18], include shortness of breath, diaphoresis, light headed-
ness, nausea and vomiting. Gender-differences exist regarding clinical presentation with typical or "atypical" angina
pectoris, which may be related to differences in pain perception in women versus men [4]. Indeed, it has been reported
that women are more likely to perceive chest pain earlier
after the onset of ischaemia, as compared with men [18].

It has also been shown that the type of pain reported by
women often has less specific features than pain reported by
men with epicardial obstructive coronary artery disease.
There is also a higher prevalence of atypical chest pain
among women compared with men, which may explain why
physicians may be less inclined to request diagnostic tests in
women compared with men [32]. The Euro Heart Survey
reported that despite a similar clinical presentation, women
were less likely than men to undergo diagnostic tests, i.e.
exercise ECG and coronary angiography [33].

Before the age of 55, the prevalence of 'atypical' and 'non-
cardiac' chest pain in women is as common as 'typical' angina
[18]. In older women, however, the prevalence of typical
angina is similar to that in men but studies have shown that
for a given degree of CAD women tend to be more symptomatic and show worse functional status than men [13].

Diagnostic Tests

Non-invasive diagnostic tests are less sensitive and specific in
women than in men, as discussed by Crea et al. [6]. Exercise

or dobutamine stress echocardiography are useful diagnostic tests in both women and men. As discussed in other chapters in the book, stress echocardiography shows regional wall motion abnormalities in subjects with ischaemia caused by epicardial coronary stenosis, but is less commonly positive in patients with microvascular angina [34].

Myocardial perfusion studies. Sensitivity and specificity of single photon emission computed tomography (SPECT) may be affected by the relatively frequent presence of artefacts, caused by smaller left ventricular chamber size and attenuation from breast tissue in women [35, 36].

Results from the WOMEN trial suggest that nuclear stress testing does not provide additional diagnostic insight in low risk women able to perform standard exercise ECG stress testing [37].

Coronary Angiography. A recent report [15] of data from the Swedish Coronary Angiography and Angioplasty Register (SCAAR), showed that non-obstructive CAD was more prevalent (78.8 % vs. 42.3 %, respectively, P 0.001) in women in the group <59 years of age. In the same age group men were more likely to have left-main stem stenosis or three-vessel disease (18.2 % vs. 4.2 %, P < 0.001). Interestingly, complication rates of coronary angiography are higher in women, and there may be a relationship between this and the fact that women have smaller coronary vessels as compared with men, despite correction for body surface area [38]. In stable CAD, a gender referral bias has been suggested to exist regarding angiography, whereby women are less likely than men to be investigated angiographically, as documented in different studies [39].

Treatment and Clinical Outcomes

Goals of treatment should be similar in men and women and recommendations from American and European guidelines have reinforced this message [40]. Of interest however, representation of women even in the latest landmark studies such as COURAGE, has been disappointing with female patients constituting only 15–30 % of the total study cohorts [41, 42].

In Europe and the USA, however, gender biases have been detected regarding the application of evidence-based treatment strategies with women who have stable angina being less likely than men to receive antiplatelet agents and lipid lowering drugs, even after the angiographic documentation of obstructive CAD [33, 43, 44].

Gender biases have been also detected regarding myocardial revascularisation. Despite the presence of angiographically documented obstructive CAD, women are less likely than men to be offered revascularisation [43]. There are also gender differences between men and women regarding the result of coronary artery bypass grafting (CABG). CABG is considered to represent the treatment of choice for significant left main coronary artery disease or triple-vessel CAD disease in patients with LV systolic dysfunction, but women who undergo CABG generally have less symptomatic relief than men [43], and this has been attributed to smaller-diameter vessels and less complete revascularisation in women.

Crea et al. [6] have elegantly discussed this topic in a recent review article. They discussed results of the 'prospeCtive observational LongitudinAl RegIstry oF patients with stable coronary arterY disease (CLARIFY)' [45], which included over 30,000 patients and showed no excess of cardiovascular events in women compared to men. However, they noted that "fewer women underwent testing and revascularisation or received optimal therapy, despite a greater burden of cardiovascular risk factors". Moreover, "among younger or lower-risk patient groups, women actually fared better than men". Andreotti and Marchese [4] indicate that "an important limitation of this and other studies is the absence of systematic angiographic data, which often reveal less extensive epicardial artery disease in women with angina compared to men". Data from the Euro Heart Survey, showed that women with angiographic CAD were less likely than men to get complete relief from angina (43 % of women being asymptomatic at follow-up, compared with 53 % of men; $P = 0.007$). Regarding major events, women were two times more likely than men to suffer death or myocardial infarction during follow-up, even after adjustment for age, abnormal LV function, diabetes, and severity or extent of CAD [43]. The same study showed that female gender was not a significant predictor of adverse outcome in the overall population with angina, but only in patients with angiographically documented CAD. Thus, Crea et al. [6] speculate that "the worse female outcome may be related to the highly selected nature of the investigated population, given the underuse of invasive imaging in women". In general, studies have shown that in unselected populations, outcomes for men and women with stable angina are generally similar, despite the fact that women may be subjected to some degree of treatment bias [6].

Outcomes of stable angina, with non-obstructive epicardial artery disease, has been discussed in other chapters in the book. Prognosis was originally thought to be excellent in these patients. A report from a registry cohort of 32,000 patients undergoing coronary angiography in Canada showed good prognosis regarding hard cardiovascular outcomes in such patients, i.e. death rate and stroke rate at 1 year follow up were 1 % and 0.6 % respectively. However, among these patients a proportion required coronary angiography due to the development of acute coronary syndromes [46].

Moreover, the Swedish Registry study [15] showed that event rates for death and rehospitalization for ischemic events, including myocardial infarction and repeat coronary angiography, were similarly low for men and women with normal or non-obstructive CAD, compared with patients with significant CAD.

Recently, however, the Women's Ischaemia Syndrome Evaluation (WISE), and other investigations, have shown that prognosis in these patients is less benign than originally thought [47, 48]. In WISE, women with reduced coronary flow reserve <2.3 had a 5-year adverse event rate of 27 %, compared with 12 % in women with CFR >2.3 (P < 0.01).

As reviewed by K. Schenck-Gustafsson [7], the prognosis of women with chest pain without obstructive CAD may be adversely impacted by the presence of concomitant coronary microvascular coronary dysfunction [49–53].

Important messages can be derived from all of the above mentioned studies, particularly that efforts should be made to risk stratify these individuals more accurately in order to identify those who are at a higher risk and require more aggressive diagnostic and therapeutic strategies.

References

1. Maas AHEM, van der Schouw YT, Regitz-Zagrosek V, Swahn E, Appelman YE, Pasterkamp G, Ten Cate H, Nilsson PM, Huisman MV, Stam HCG, Eizema K, Stramba-Badiale M. Red alert for women's heart: the urgent need for more research and knowledge on cardiovascular disease in women: proceedings of the workshop held in Brussels on gender differences in cardiovascular disease, 29 September 2010. Eur Heart J. 2011;32:1362–8.

2. Stramba-Badiale M, Fox KM, Priori SG, Collins P, Daly C, Graham I, Jonsson B, Schenck-Gustafsson K, Tendera M. Cardiovascular diseases in women: a statement from the policy conference of the European Society of Cardiology. Eur Heart J. 2006;27:994–1005.

3. Rosamond W, Flegal K, Friday G, Furie K, Go A, Greenlund K, Haase N, Ho M, Howard V, Kissela B, Kissela B, Kittner S, Lloyd-Jones D, McDermott M, Meigs J, Moy C, Nichol G, O'Donnell CJ, Roger V, Rumsfeld J, Sorlie P, Steinberger J, Thom T, Wasserthiel-Smoller S, Hong Y, American Heart Association Statistics Committee and Stroke Statistics Subcommittee. Heart disease and stroke statistics – 2007 update: a report from the American Heart Association Statistics Committee and Stroke Statistics Subcommittee. Circulation. 2007;115:e69–171.

4. Andreotti F, Marchese N. Women and coronary disease. Heart. 2008;94:108–16.

5. National Institutes of Health. National Heart, Lung, and Blood Institute, Incidence and prevalence: 2006 chart book on cardiovascular and lung diseases. Bethesda; 2006.

6. Crea F, Battipaglia I, Andreotti F. Sex differences in mechanisms, presentation and management of ischaemic heart disease. Atherosclerosis. 2015;241:157–68.

7. Schenck-Gustafsson K. Angina in women: epidemiology, prognosis and diagnosis. In: Kaski JC, Eslick GD, Bairey Merz CN, editors. Chest pain with normal coronary arteries – a multidisciplinary approach. London: Springer; 2013.

8. Murabito JM, Evans JC, Larson MG, Levy D. Prognosis after the onset of coronary heart disease. An investigation of differences in outcome between the sexes according to initial coronary disease presentation. Circulation. 1993;88:2548–55.

9. World Health Statistics. Chapter 2: cause-specific mortality and morbidity. 2012. www.who.int/whosis.

10. Hemingway H, Langenberg C, Damant J, Frost C, Pyörälä K, Barrett-Connor E. Prevalence of angina in women versus men: a systematic review and meta-analysis of international variations across 31 countries. Circulation. 2008;117:1526–36.

11. Hemingway H, McCallum A, Shipley M, Manderbacka K, Martikainen P, Keskimaki I. Incidence and prognostic implications of stable angina pectoris among women and men. JAMA. 2006;295:1404–11.

12. Shaw LJ, Shaw RE, Merz CNB, Brindis RG, Klein LW, Nallamothu B, Douglas PS, Krone RJ, McKay CR, Block PC, Hewitt K, Weintraub WS, Peterson ED, American College of Cardiology-National Cardiovascular Data Registry Investigators. Impact of ethnicity and gender differences on angiographic coronary artery disease prevalence and in-hospital mortality in the American College of Cardiology-National Cardiovascular Data Registry. Circulation. 2008;117:1787–801.

13. Davis KB, Chaitman B, Ryan T, Bittner V, Kennedy JW. Comparison of 15-year survival for men and women after initial medical or surgical treatment for coronary artery disease: a CASS registry study. Coronary Artery Surgery Study. J Am Coll Cardiol. 1995;25:1000–9.

14. Shaw LJ, Merz CNB, Pepine CJ, Reis SE, Bittner V, Kip KE, Kelsey SF, Olson M, Johnson BD, Mankad S, Sharaf BL, Rogers WJ, Pohost GM, Sopko G, Women's Ischemia Syndrome Evaluation (WISE) Investigators. The economic burden of angina in women with suspected ischemic heart disease: results from the National Institutes of Health – National Heart, Lung, and Blood Institute – sponsored Women's Ischemia Syndrome Evaluation. Circulation. 2006;114:894–904.

15. Johnston N, Schenck-Gustafsson K, Lagerqvist B. Are we using cardiovascular medications and coronary angiography

appropriately in men and women with chest pain? Eur Heart J. 2011;32:1331–6.

16. Rosamond W, Flegal K, Furie K, Go A, Greenlund K, Haase N, Hailpern SM, Ho M, Howard V, Kissela B, Kissela B, Kittner S, Lloyd-Jones D, McDermott M, Meigs J, Moy C, Nichol G, O'Donnell C, Roger V, Sorlie P, Steinberger J, Thom T, Wilson M, Hong Y, American Heart Association Statistics Committee and Stroke Statistics Subcommittee. Heart disease and stroke statistics – 2008 update: a report from the American Heart Association Statistics Committee and Stroke Statistics Subcommittee. Circulation. 2008;117:e25–146.

17. Mosca L, Benjamin EJ, Berra K, Bezanson JL, Dolor RJ, Lloyd-Jones DM, Newby LK, Piña IL, Roger VL, Shaw LJ, Zhao D, Beckie TM, Bushnell C, D'Armiento J, Kris-Etherton PM, Fang J, Ganiats TG, Gomes AS, Gracia CR, Haan CK, Jackson EA, Judelson DR, Kelepouris E, Lavie CJ, Moore A, Nussmeier NA, Ofili E, Oparil S, Ouyang P, Pinn VW, et al. Effectiveness-based guidelines for the prevention of cardiovascular disease in women – 2011 update: a guideline from the american heart association. Circulation. 2011;123:1243–62.

18. Shaw LJ, Bairey Merz CN, Pepine CJ, Reis SE, Bittner V, Kelsey SF, Olson M, Johnson BD, Mankad S, Sharaf BL, Rogers WJ, Wessel TR, Arant CB, Pohost GM, Lerman A, Quyyumi AA, Sopko G, WISE Investigators. Insights from the NHLBI-Sponsored Women's Ischemia Syndrome Evaluation (WISE) Study: part I: gender differences in traditional and novel risk factors, symptom evaluation, and gender-optimized diagnostic strategies. J Am Coll Cardiol. 2006;47:S4–20.

19. Hsia J, Aragaki A, Bloch M, LaCroix AZ, Wallace R, Investigators WHI. Predictors of angina pectoris versus myocardial infarction from the Women's Health Initiative Observational Study. Am J Cardiol. 2004;93:673–8.

20. World Health Organization. Economic costs. 2000. http://www.who.int/cardiovascular_diseases/en/cvd_atlas_17_economics.pdf. 1 Aug 2012.

21. Johnson BD, Shaw LJ, Pepine CJ, Reis SE, Kelsey SF, Sopko G, Rogers WJ, Mankad S, Sharaf BL, Bittner V, Bairey Merz CN. Persistent chest pain predicts cardiovascular events in women without obstructive coronary artery disease: results from the NIH-NHLBI-sponsored Women's Ischaemia Syndrome Evaluation (WISE) study. Eur Heart J. 2006;27:1408–15.

22. Mozaffarian D, Benjamin EJ, Go AS, Arnett DK, Blaha MJ, Cushman M, de Ferranti S, Després J-P, Fullerton HJ, Howard VJ, Huffman MD, Judd SE, Kissela BM, Lackland DT, Lichtman JH, Lisabeth LD, Liu S, Mackey RH, Matchar DB, McGuire DK, Mohler ER, Moy CS, Muntner P, Mussolino ME, Nasir K, Neumar RW, Nichol G, Palaniappan L, Pandey DK, Reeves MJ, et al. Heart disease and stroke statistics – 2015 update: a report from the American Heart Association. Circulation. 2015; 131:e29–322.

23. Huxley R, Barzi F, Woodward M. Excess risk of fatal coronary heart disease associated with diabetes in men and women: meta-analysis of 37 prospective cohort studies. BMJ. 2006;332:73–8.

24. Preis SR, Hwang S-J, Coady S, Pencina MJ, D'Agostino RB, Savage PJ, Levy D, Fox CS. Trends in all-cause and cardiovascular disease mortality among women and men with and without diabetes mellitus in the Framingham Heart Study, 1950 to 2005. Circulation. 2009;119:1728–35.

25. Regitz-Zagrosek V, Lehmkuhl E, Mahmoodzadeh S. Gender aspects of the role of the metabolic syndrome as a risk factor for cardiovascular disease. Gend Med. 2007;4 Suppl B:S162–77.

26. Anand SS, Islam S, Rosengren A, Franzosi MG, Steyn K, Yusufali AH, Keltai M, Diaz R, Rangarajan S, Yusuf S, INTERHEART Investigators. Risk factors for myocardial infarction in women and men: insights from the INTERHEART study. Eur Heart J. 2008;29:932–40.

27. The decline of ischaemic heart disease mortality in the ARIC study communities. The ARIC Study Investigators. Int J Epidemiol. 1989;18:S88–98.

28. Kannel WB, Feinleib M. Natural history of angina pectoris in the Framingham study. Prognosis and survival. Am J Cardiol. 1972;29:154–63.

29. Ferrari R, Abergel H, Ford I, Fox KM, Greenlaw N, Steg PG, Hu D, Tendera M, Tardif J-C, CLARIFY Investigators. Gender- and age-related differences in clinical presentation and management of outpatients with stable coronary artery disease. Int J Cardiol. 2013;167:2938–43.

30. Lerner DJ, Kannel WB. Patterns of coronary heart disease morbidity and mortality in the sexes: a 26-year follow-up of the Framingham population. Am Heart J. 1986;111:383–90.

31. Reunanen A, Suhonen O, Aromaa A, Knekt P, Pyörälä K. Incidence of different manifestations of coronary heart

disease in middle-aged Finnish men and women. Acta Med Scand. 1985;218:19–26.

32. Vaccarino V, Krumholz HM, Yarzebski J, Gore JM, Goldberg RJ. Sex differences in 2-year mortality after hospital discharge for myocardial infarction. Ann Intern Med. 2001;134:173–81.

33. Schenck-Gustafsson K. Coronary heart disease. In: Schenck-Gustafsson K, DeCola PR, Pfaff DW, Pisetsky D, editors. Handbook of clinical gender medicine. Basel: Karger Verlag; 2012. p. 190–2005.

34. Montalescot G, Sechtem U, Achenbach S, Andreotti F, Arden C, Budaj A, Bugiardini R, Crea F, Cuisset T, Di Mario C, Ferreira JR, Gersh BJ, Gitt AK, Hulot JS, Marx N, Opie LH, Pfisterer M, Prescott E, Ruschitzka F, Sabaté M, Senior R, Taggart DP, Van Der Wall EE, Vrints CJM, Zamorano JL, Baumgartner H, Bax JJ, Bueno H, Dean V, Deaton C, et al. 2013 ESC guidelines on the management of stable coronary artery disease. Eur Heart J. 2013;34:2949–3003.

35. Fleischmann KE, Hunink MG, Kuntz KM, Douglas PS. Exercise echocardiography or exercise SPECT imaging? A meta-analysis of diagnostic test performance. JAMA. 1998;280:913–20.

36. Duvall WL. Cardiovascular disease in women. Mt Sinai J Med. 2003;70:293–305.

37. Shaw LJ, Mieres JH, Hendel RH, Boden WE, Gulati M, Veledar E, Hachamovitch R, Arrighi JA, Merz CNB, Gibbons RJ, Wenger NK, Heller GV, WOMEN Trial Investigators. Comparative effectiveness of exercise electrocardiography with or without myocardial perfusion single photon emission computed tomography in women with suspected coronary artery disease: results from the What Is the Optimal Method for Ischemia Evaluation in Women (WOMEN) trial. Circulation. 2011;124:1239–49.

38. Kitzman DW, Scholz DG, Hagen PT, Ilstrup DM, Edwards WD. Age-related changes in normal human hearts during the first 10 decades of life. Part II (Maturity): a quantitative anatomic study of 765 specimens from subjects 20 to 99 years old. Mayo Clin Proc. 1988;63:137–46.

39. Daly CA, Clemens F, Sendon JLL, Tavazzi L, Boersma E, Danchin N, Delahaye F, Gitt A, Julian D, Mulcahy D, Ruzyllo W, Thygesen K, Verheugt F, Fox KM, Euro Heart Survey Investigators. The clinical characteristics and investigations planned in patients with stable angina presenting to cardiologists in Europe: from the Euro Heart Survey of Stable Angina. Eur Heart J. 2005;26:996–1010.

40. Zellweger MJ, Pfisterer ME. Therapeutic strategies in patients with chronic stable coronary artery disease. Cardiovasc Ther. 2011;29:e23–30.

41. Boden WE, O'Rourke RA, Teo KK, Hartigan PM, Maron DJ, Kostuk WJ, Knudtson M, Dada M, Casperson P, Harris CL, Chaitman BR, Shaw L, Gosselin G, Nawaz S, Title LM, Gau G, Blaustein AS, Booth DC, Bates ER, Spertus JA, Berman DS, Mancini GBJ, Weintraub WS, COURAGE Trial Research Group. Optimal medical therapy with or without PCI for stable coronary disease. N Engl J Med. 2007;356:1503–16.

42. BARI 2D Study Group, Frye RL, August P, Brooks MM, Hardison RM, Kelsey SF, MacGregor JM, Orchard TJ, Chaitman BR, Genuth SM, Goldberg SH, Hlatky MA, Jones TLZ, Molitch ME, Nesto RW, Sako EY, Sobel BE. A randomized trial of therapies for type 2 diabetes and coronary artery disease. N Engl J Med. 2009;360:2503–15.

43. Daly C, Clemens F, Lopez Sendon JL, Tavazzi L, Boersma E, Danchin N, Delahaye F, Gitt A, Julian D, Mulcahy D, Ruzyllo W, Thygesen K, Verheugt F, Fox KM, Euro Heart Survey Investigators. Gender differences in the management and clinical outcome of stable angina. Circulation. 2006;113:490–8.

44. Bickell NA, Pieper KS, Lee KL, Mark DB, Glower DD, Pryor DB, Califf RM. Referral patterns for coronary artery disease treatment: gender bias or good clinical judgment? Ann Intern Med. 1992;116:791–7.

45. Steg PG, Greenlaw N, Tardif J-C, Tendera M, Ford I, Kääb S, Abergel H, Fox KM, Ferrari R, CLARIFY Registry Investigators. Women and men with stable coronary artery disease have similar clinical outcomes: insights from the international prospective CLARIFY registry. Eur Heart J. 2012;33:2831–40.

46. Humphries KH, Pu A, Gao M, Carere RG, Pilote L. Angina with 'normal' coronary arteries: sex differences in outcomes. Am Heart J. 2008;155:375–81.

47. Pepine CJ, Anderson RD, Sharaf BL, Reis SE, Smith KM, Handberg EM, Johnson BD, Sopko G, Bairey Merz CN. Coronary microvascular reactivity to adenosine predicts adverse outcome in women evaluated for suspected ischemia results from the National Heart, Lung and Blood Institute WISE (Women's Ischemia Syndrome Evaluation) study. J Am Coll Cardiol. 2010;55:2825–32.

48. Gulati M, Cooper-DeHoff RM, McClure C, Johnson BD, Shaw LJ, Handberg EM, Zineh I, Kelsey SF, Arnsdorf MF, Black HR,

Pepine CJ, Merz CNB. Adverse cardiovascular outcomes in women with nonobstructive coronary artery disease: a report from the Women's Ischemia Syndrome Evaluation Study and the St James Women Take Heart Project. Arch Intern Med. 2009;169:843–50.

49. Hurst T, Olson TH, Olson LE, Appleton CP. Cardiac syndrome X and endothelial dysfunction: new concepts in prognosis and treatment. Am J Med. 2006;119:560–6.

50. Doyle M, Fuisz A, Kortright E, Biederman RW, Walsh EG, Martin ET, Tauxe L, Rogers WJ, Merz CN, Pepine C, Sharaf B, Pohost GM. The impact of myocardial flow reserve on the detection of coronary artery disease by perfusion imaging methods: an NHLBI WISE study. J Cardiovasc Magn Reson. 2003;5:475–85.

51. Reis SE, Holubkov R, Lee JS, Sharaf B, Reichek N, Rogers WJ, Walsh EG, Fuisz AR, Kerensky R, Detre KM, Sopko G, Pepine CJ. Coronary flow velocity response to adenosine characterizes coronary microvascular function in women with chest pain and no obstructive coronary disease. Results from the pilot phase of the Women's Ischemia Syndrome Evaluation (WISE) study. J Am Coll Cardiol. 1999;33:1469–75.

52. Suwaidi JA, Hamasaki S, Higano ST, Nishimura RA, Holmes DR, Lerman A. Long-term follow-up of patients with mild coronary artery disease and endothelial dysfunction. Circulation. 2000;101:948–54.

53. Bugiardini R, Bairey Merz CN. Angina with 'normal' coronary arteries: a changing philosophy. JAMA. 2005;293:477–84.

Chapter 6
Management of Angina

Abstract Chronic stable angina caused by coronary artery disease is not only a very frequent condition, but it is also associated with an increased risk of major cardiovascular events. There are other important mechanisms of angina pectoris involving coronary microvascular dysfunction and reduced coronary blood flow reserve. Once the diagnosis of angina is confirmed, and the mechanisms responsible for myocardial ischaemia identified, treatment should be started without delay. The key objectives of the treatment of angina pectoris in both coronary disease patients and patients with microvascular angina include improve symptoms and quality of life as well as clinical outcomes such as mortality and major cardiovascular events. The bulk of the evidence regarding the effects of risk factor management, lifestyle changes and preventative pharmacological therapy in angina pectoris, has been gathered in patients suffering from obstructive coronary artery disease. Lesser information, however, is available regarding interventions that affect prognosis in microvascular angina. International guidelines recommend lifestyle changes, aggressive risk factor management and the use of pharmacological agents as well as coronary intervention when indicated. This chapter discusses the various options available for management of this common condition.

Introduction

As recently reviewed by Ohman in the *New England Journal of Medicine* [1] and as mentioned in previous chapters in this book, chronic stable angina pectoris is a common manifestation of coronary artery disease, with approximately seven million

American people suffering from angina [2]. Chronic stable angina caused by coronary artery disease is not only a very frequent condition, but it is also associated with an increased risk of major cardiovascular events [3, 4]. Studies have reported that patients with angina very often have risk factors and/or comorbidities, which are commonly associated with an increased risk of myocardial infarction and cardiovascular death. Among these advanced age, chronic kidney disease, diabetes, heart failure, and a markedly reduced exercise capacity feature prominently [5, 6]. Of importance, chronic stable angina represents a substantial financial burden to health systems Worldwide and may have a major financial impact on many of the individuals affected by the condition [7].

Another relatively common form of angina pectoris, as discussed in other chapters of this book, is "microvascular angina" – also known as "cardiac syndrome X" [8–10]

Patients with microvascular angina have an impaired quality of life as a result of frequent and prolonged episodes of chest pain. Prognosis can be impaired in these patients, particularly in those found to have a markedly abnormal coronary flow reserve [11–13],

Once the diagnosis of angina is confirmed, treatment should be started without delay. It is important, however, to establish a clear therapeutic strategy tailored to the individual patient. Guidelines from the ESC [14], as well as those from NICE [15] and the ACC/AHA [16], are extremely helpful for this purpose.

This chapter will focus mainly on the pharmacological management of angina. Content in this monographic work is based on current recommendations by the ESC and AHA/ACC for the management of stable angina pectoris.

Objectives of Treatment

The key objectives of the treatment of angina pectoris in both coronary disease patients and patients with microvascular angina are: (1) To improve symptoms and quality of life and (2) To improve clinical outcomes i.e. mortality and major cardiovascular events [14, 16, 17].

General Principles of Treatment

Most of the therapeutic interventions suggested in this section should be used for managing both typical angina caused by obstructive coronary artery disease and microvascular angina patients. The bulk of the evidence, however, regarding the effects of risk factor management, lifestyle changes and preventative pharmacological therapy in angina pectoris, has been gathered in patients suffering from obstructive coronary artery disease. Less information is available regarding interventions that affect prognosis in microvascular angina, albeit the consensus at present is that risk factor modification and lifestyle changes are also likely to be beneficial in the management of microvascular angina. This chapter is based on the recommendations of the ESC guidelines for the management of stable angina pectoris [14] and also incorporates recommendations by the AHA/ACC guidelines [16].

Management of Typical Angina Pectoris Caused by Obstructive Coronary Artery Disease

Risk Factor Management and Lifestyle Changes

Lifestyle is important and evidence based lifestyle changes should be strongly recommended to all patients, as appropriate. These include weight loss in overweight or obese patients, dietary changes to reduce fat and sugar intake, exercise and smoking cessation.

Weight Management

Clinical diagnoses of obesity, or being overweight, are associated with an increased risk of death in patients with coronary artery disease. Weight reduction in overweight patients has been shown to have beneficial effects on blood pressure, dyslipidaemia and the metabolic syndrome [18] In obese patients it is important to assess whether sleep apnoea is present, as this condition has been associated with increased cardiovascular mortality and morbidity [19].

Diet

A healthy diet reduces cardiovascular risk. Dietary energy intake should be limited to that suitable to reach or maintain a BMI <25 kg/m^2. N-3 polyunsaturated fatty acid (PUFA) consumption is recommended but mainly from oily fish in the diet without the need for supplements. PUFA intake has been associated with beneficial actions on cardiac risk factors in some studies but this is not a universal finding [20–22]. The 'Mediterranean' diet, supplemented with extra-virgin olive oil or nuts, has been shown to reduce major cardiovascular events in patients at high risk [23].

Lipid Management

Dyslipidaemia should be managed according to lipid guidelines, which recommend a combination of pharmacological intervention and lifestyle changes [24]. As recommended by the ESC guidelines, patients with coronary artery disease should receive treatment with statins, irrespective of low density lipoprotein (LDL) cholesterol (LDL-C) levels. Treatment targets have been set at LDL-C <1.8 mmol/L (<70 mg/dL) or >50 % LDL-C reduction when the target level cannot be achieved. Fibrates, nicotinic acid and ezetimibe may also lower LDL cholesterol but these agents do not appear to affect clinical outcomes. For patients undergoing percutaneous coronary intervention (PCI) for stable coronary artery disease, high dose atorvastatin has been shown to reduce the incidence of peri-procedural myocardial infarction [24, 25]. Randomised, placebo-controlled trials have suggested that high-intensity statins that reduce LDL cholesterol levels by >50 % can also decrease daily episodes of angina [26] and improve exercise tolerance [27] in patients with chronic stable angina who are already receiving antianginal therapy.

Furthermore, a randomized trial comparing high intensity statin therapy with PCI in patients with stable coronary artery disease showed a lower rate of ischemic cardiac events (non-significant) among patients who received atorvastatin therapy compared to the PCI group [28].

Smoking

Smoking is a strong independent risk factor for cardiovascular disease and there is a clear recommendation in all guidelines that all forms of smoking be discontinued/avoided in patients with coronary disease [29]. The benefits of smoking cessation are established [30], and smoking cessation is associated with a reduction in mortality of 36 % after myocardial infarction [31]. It is recommended that smoking status (all forms, including passive smoking) should be assessed systematically in every coronary artery disease patient and smokers strongly advised to quit [18]. Pharmacological agents can help patients to quit smoking and it has been shown that nicotine replacement therapy is safe in patients with coronary artery disease [32, 33]. Currently available pharmacological agents (i.e. bupropion and varenicline) have also been found to be safe in patients with stable coronary artery disease, albeit the safety of varenicline has been questioned recently [34].

Physical Activity

Physical activity can reduce morbidity and mortality in patients with coronary artery disease. Aerobic exercise should be offered to patients with known coronary artery disease, within a structured cardiac rehabilitation programme. It has been recommended that patients with a previous acute myocardial infarction, by-pass surgery, PCI, stable angina pectoris or stable chronic heart failure should undergo aerobic exercise training ≥3 times a week and for 30 min per session.

Arterial Hypertension

Elevated blood pressure is a major risk factor for coronary artery disease, heart failure, cerebrovascular disease and renal failure. Systolic blood pressure should be lowered to <140 mmHg and diastolic pressure to <90 mmHg in stable angina patients with hypertension. The ESC guidelines recommend to lower blood pressure to values within the range 130–139/80–85 mmHg [18, 35]. Recent data from SPRINT suggest that attempts should be made to reduce blood pressure to below 120/85 mmHg [36], albeit changes to guideline recommendations are unlikely to occur in the immediate future.

Diabetes

Diabetes mellitus is a strong risk factor for cardiovascular events and increases the risk of coronary disease progression. Good control of glycated haemoglobin (HbA1c), i.e. <7.0 % (53 mmol/mol) on average and <6.5 %–6.9 % (48–52 mmol/mol) in the individual patient, is recommended by International guidelines. Of interest, the "traditional" goal for blood pressure management in diabetes, i.e. <130 mmHg, is not supported by evidence in outcome trials. Based on this, ESC guidelines recommend a blood pressure target <140/85 mmHg and the administration of angiotensin converting enzyme (ACE) inhibitors or renin-angiotensin receptor blockers in patients with diabetes and coronary artery disease [18, 37, 38].

Chronic Kidney Disease (CKD)

CKD patients are at high risk of developing cardiovascular events and require intensive management of all risk factors, particularly hypertension and dyslipidaemia.

Hormone Replacement Therapy (HRT)

Results from large randomised trials do not support the use of HRT for primary or secondary prevention of cardiovascular disease [39].

Preventative Pharmacological Measures with an Impact on Outcome

Several preventative therapies have been shown to be effective and should therefore be started without delay in patients with coronary disease [14, 16].

Aspirin and Other Antiplatelet Agents

Antiplatelet agents decrease platelet aggregation and prevent coronary thrombus formation. Due to a favourable ratio between benefit and risk in patients with stable CAD, and its low cost, low-dose aspirin ($\geq$75 mg/day) is the drug of choice in most cases. Aspirin acts via irreversible inhibition of platelet cyclooxygenase-1 (COX-1) and reduces thromboxane production [40–42].

A meta-analysis of primary-prevention trials showed that the rate of cardiovascular events was 18 % lower among people taking aspirin than among controls ($p < 0.001$). Aspirin reduced the rate of myocardial infarction by 23 %. Aspirin did not, however, have a significant effect on the rate of death from cardiovascular causes. Compared with controls, patients who took aspirin had similar rates of intracranial bleeding, but higher rates of gastrointestinal bleeding [43].

P2Y12 Inhibitors

P2Y12 inhibitors, including thienopyridines, act as antagonists of the platelet adenosine diphosphate (ADP) receptor inhibiting platelet aggregation. The largest study supporting the use of thienopyridines in stable coronary patients is the Clopidogrel vs. Aspirin in Patients at Risk of Ischaemic Events (CAPRIE) trial. CAPRIE showed an overall benefit of clopidogrel over aspirin for prevention of cardiovascular events in patients with previous myocardial infarction, previous stroke or peripheral vascular disease (PVD) [44]. Importantly, the benefits of clopidogrel were mainly driven by effects seen in patients with PVD. ESC guidelines recommend considering clopidogrel as a second-line treatment, especially for aspirin-intolerant CVD patients. Prasugrel and ticagrelor are new P2Yantagonists that achieve greater platelet inhibition, compared with clopidogrel [45, 46]. Prasugrel and ticagrelor are both associated with a significant reduction of cardiovascular outcomes, compared with clopidogrel in ACS patients [47, 48], but no clinical studies have evaluated the effects of these drugs in chronic stable angina patients.

Regarding dual antiplatelet therapy in stable angina, in the Clopidogrel for High Atherothrombotic Risk and Ischemic Stabilization, Management, and Avoidance (CHARISMA) study [49], dual antiplatelet therapy was of no benefit in patients with stable vascular disease or those at risk of developing atherothrombotic events. A significant benefit was observed however in a post-hoc analysis of patients with documented atherothrombotic disease and in patients with a prior history of myocardial infarction [50].

Lipid-Lowering Agents (See section "Lipid Management")

Patients with documented coronary disease are at high risk of events and should receive treatment with statins, as recommended by the ESC/European Atherosclerosis Society Guidelines for the management of dyslipidaemia [24]. The recommended treatment target is LDL-C <1.8 mmol/L or >50 % reduction in LDL-C when the target level cannot be achieved.

Angiotensin-Converting Enzyme Inhibitors

The European guidelines for the management of stable IHD (2013) [14] recommend the use of angiotensin-converting enzyme inhibitors (ACEi) for event prevention in patients with stable coronary artery disease, particularly in the presence of comorbidities such as heart failure, hypertension, or diabetes. Angiotensin Receptor Blockers (ARBs) may be an alternative therapy but only when ACEi are not tolerated. Currently, there are no clinical outcome studies showing a beneficial effect of ARBs in stable coronary artery disease patients [14] . The ACEi perindopril has been shown, in more than 12,000 patients with coronary artery disease included in the EUROPA study, to significantly reduce CV mortality by 20 %, fatal and non-fatal MI by 25 %, and hospitalization for heart failure by 39 % [51].

EUROPA trial was designed to assess whether the ACEi perindopril could reduce cardiovascular risk in a relatively low-risk population with stable coronary heart disease and no clini-cally apparent heart failure. 13,655 patients – mean age 60 years, 85 % men – were recruited in the period from October 1997 to June 2000. Of these, a history of previous myocardial infarction was present in 64 % and angiographic evidence of coronary artery disease was obtained in 61 %. Fifty-five percent had undergone coronary revascularisation. After a run-in period of 4 weeks, in which all patients received perindopril, 12,218 patients were randomly assigned to perindopril 8 mg once daily (n = 6110), or matching placebo (n = 6108). The mean follow-up time was 4.2 years, and the primary endpoint was cardiovascu-lar death, myocardial infarction, or cardiac arrest.

Main findings in the study were as follow: 92 % were taking platelet inhibitors, 62 % beta-blockers, and 58 % lipid-lowering therapy. Six hundred and three (10 %) of patients receiving pla-cebo and 488 (8 %) patients on perindopril experienced the primary endpoint, which represents a 20 % relative risk reduc-tion (95 % CI 9–29, p = 0.0003) associated with the administra-tion of perindopril. Of importance, these benefits were consistent in all predefined patient subgroups. Findings in this important study involving patients with stable coronary heart disease with-out heart failure, indicate that perindopril can improve patient clinical outcomes even in individuals who are at an intermediate risk of developing cardiovascular events. Based on the results of this study, current guidelines recommend the use of ACEi, i.e. perindopril, in addition to all other preventative treatments, in patients with coronary heart disease.

The beneficial effects observed in the EUROPA trial [51] have been further highlighted in a recent review published by Strauss and Hall, suggesting divergent cardiovascular effects of ACEi compared with ARBs, particularly in terms of reduction in risk of myocardial infarction and total mortality in high risk hypertensive patients [52].

Beta-blockers, which are discussed later in this chapter, reduce heart rate, contractility, atrioventricular conduction and ectopic activity. Additionally, they may increase perfusion of ischemic areas by prolonging diastolic time and slightly increasing vascular resistance in non-ischemic areas. A recent sub-analysis of EUROPA trial including 7534 patients taking a beta-blocking agent at baseline showed a significant reduction in fatal and non-fatal MI (28 % reduction) and in the composite primary outcome (24 %) including cardiovascular death, nonfatal myocardial infarction, and cardiac arrest. A larger reduction (45 %) was observed regarding hospitalization for heart failure when perindopril and beta-blockers were compared with a combination of placebo and beta-blockers. Findings in this study indicate that the addition of perindopril to beta-blockers in stable coronary artery disease patients was safe and resulted in improved cardiovascular outcomes and mortality rates compared with standard therapies, including beta-blockers [53].

Symptomatic Therapies for Angina

General Considerations

Antianginal therapy should be initiated as soon as possible after the diagnosis of angina has been made. The goal of antianginal therapy is to reduce both symptoms and exercise-induced ischemia [54]. Sublingual nitrates should be prescribed to all patients with suspected angina and patients should be carefully instructed as to when and how to use these agents. Long-term antianginal therapies should also be initiated, as suggested by Husted and Ohman, "with attention to the patient's resting heart rate and blood pressure" [54]. A suggested approach for the use of various types of antianginal therapies is shown in Fig. 6.1.

Standard Antianginal Therapies

The choice of initial antianginal therapy should be tailored to the individual, taking into account the specific goals of therapy in a given patient, patient comorbidities, and drug characteristics and side effects. Guidelines have recommended that the most appropriate medical therapy is a combination of two antianginal agents in different drug classes: i.e. beta-blockers, calcium-channel blockers, or long-acting nitrates [14, 16].

Doses of antianginal therapies should be increased, as needed, to achieve symptom control and improvements in heart rate and blood-pressure levels. If symptoms are not relieved within 2 weeks after the initiation of therapy, coronary arteriography may be indicated (Fig. 6.2).

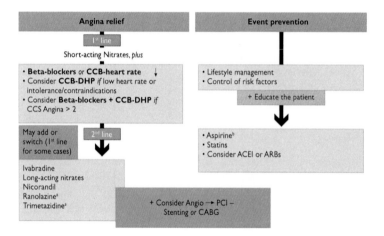

FIGURE 6.1 Medical management of patients with stable coronary artery disease (From Ref. [14] with permission). Abbreviations: *ACEI* angiotensin converting enzyme inhibitor, *CABG* coronary artery bypass graft, *CCB* calcium channel blockers, *CCS* Canadian Cardiovascular Society, *DHP* dihydropyridine, *PCI* percutaneous coronary intervention

[a]Data for diabetics

[b]If intolerance, consider clopidogrel

Indication	Class[a]	Level[b]
General considerations		
Optimal medical treatment indicates at least one drug for angina/ischaemia relief plus drug for event prevention.	I	C
It is recommended to educate patients about the disease,risk factors and treatment strategy.	I	C
It is indicated to review the patient's response soon after starting therapy.	I	C
Angina/ischaemia[c] relief		
Short-acting nitrates are recommended.	I	B
Firest-line treatment is indicated with β-blockers and/or calcium channel blockers to control heart rate and symptoms.	I	A
For second-line treatment ti is recommended to add long-acting nitrates or ivabradine or nicorandil or ranolazine, according to heart rate, blood pressure and tolerance.	IIa	B
For second-line treatment, trimetazidine may be considered.	IIb	B
According to comorbidities/tolerance it is indicated to use second-line therapies as first-line treatment in selected patients.	I	C
In asymptomatic patients with large areas of ischaemia (>10 %) β-blockers should be considered.	IIa	C
In patients with vasospastic angina,calcium chanel blockers and nitrates should be considered and beta-blockers avoided.	IIa	B
Event prevention		
Low-dose aspirin daily is recommended in all SCAD patients.	I	A
Clopidogrel is indicated as an alternative in case of aspirin intolerance.	I	B
Statins are recommended in all SCAD patients.	I	A
It is recommended to use ACE inhibitors (or ARBs) if presence of other conditions (e.g. heart failure, hypertension or diabetes).	I	A

FIGURE 6.2 Pharmacological treatments in stable coronary artery disease patients (From Ref. [14] with permission). *ACE* angiotensin converting enzyme, *SCAD* stable coronary artery disease
[a]Class of recommendation
[b]Level of evidence
[c]No demonstration of benefit on prognosis

Nitrates

Nitrates are arterial and venous vasodilators and are useful for the symptomatic relief of effort angina, acting via their active component nitric oxide (NO). Nitrates increase coronary blood flow and reduce both afterload and preload, thus decreasing myocardial oxygen consumption. Sublingual nitroglycerin is the standard initial therapy for effort induced angina. It is important that at onset of therapy patients are instructed to sit down while applying the sublingual treatment. If they remain in the standing position severe postural hypotension may develop leading to a syncopal episode. Sublingual nitroglycerin (0.3–0.6 mg) (spray or tablets) can be administered every 5 min until the pain is relieved, or a maximum dose of 1.2 mg has been taken within 15 min. Patients may be advised to use nitroglycerin "prophylactically" prior to undertaking activities known to trigger angina.

Sublingual isosorbide dinitrate (5 mg) is also effective but has a slower onset of action compared with nitroglycerin due to the hepatic conversion of the dinitrate molecule to mononitrate, required for its anti-anginal action.

Oral nitrates have longer lasting haemodynamic effects than sublingual nitrates and may offer more prolonged antianginal protection than sublingual agents [55]. Tolerance, however, may develop with the use of long-acting nitrates if they are administered over prolonged periods and without a nitrate-free interval of 8–10 h. In a large multicentre study, the extended-release formulation of isosorbide dinitrate, 40 mg given twice-daily, was not superior to placebo. Moreover, worsening of endothelial dysfunction has also been reported with the use of these agents. Taken together, these data indicate that long-acting nitrates may not represent first line therapy for patients with effort angina and that the widespread use of isosorbide dinitrate in current clinical practice is not evidence-based [15, 55]. Mononitrates have similar effects to those of isosorbide dinitrate and similar problems regarding nitrate tolerance which may be overcome at least partially by timing of administration and the use of slow-release preparations. The twice-daily use of rapid-release preparations and high dose slow-release mononitrate may give sustained anti-anginal benefit [56, 57]. Transdermal nitroglycerin patches may be useful in selected patients but little information is available from large trials.

Nitrate drug interactions should be taken into account when prescribing these agents. Hypotension may develop when used together with calcium channel blockers and very serious hypotension can occur if used together with selective PDE5 inhibitors, often prescribed for the management of erectile dysfunction or the treatment of pulmonary hypertension.

Beta-Blockers

Beta-blockers are considered to represent first line therapy for angina partly because of historical data indicating a reduction in mortality when they are administered after myocardial infarction and partly as a result of relatively old trials showing improved symptoms and exercise capacity. Regarding the former, however, two observational studies showed no significant association between beta-blocker use and mortality among patients with chronic coronary artery disease, although a reduced risk of recurrent myocardial infarction was reported with beta-blocker use [58, 59].

The TIBET (Total Ischaemic Burden European Trial) study showed that atenolol produced similar anti-anginal benefits when compared to slow-release nifedipine; no significant additional benefits were seen when the two agents were combined [60].

The most widely used beta-blockers in Europe are those exerting predominantly a blockade of the beta-1 receptor i.e. metoprolol [61], bisoprolol, atenolol and nevibolol. All of these, together with carvedilol, reduce cardiac events in patients with heart failure [62–65].

Calcium Channel Blockers

Calcium channel blockers act on L-type Ca2+ receptors and lead to systemic and coronary vasodilatation, reducing afterload and improving myocardial blood flow. Calcium channel blockers are broadly grouped under two categories: non-dihydropyridine agents and the dihydropyridine. Calcium channel blockers belonging to the non-dihydropyridine group, i.e. verapamil and diltiazem, have vasodilatory actions that reduce peripheral vascular resistance and these agents also reduce heart rate via nodal inhibition. Verapamil has many indications in cardiovascular medicine and is generally well tolerated albeit heart block, bradycardia and mild negative inotropic actions have been described. Its anti-anginal action is similar to that of metoprolol [61] and slightly superior to that of atenolol [66]. Verapamil should not be used in conjunction with beta-blockers as this combination increases the risk of heart block. Diltiazem is an effective anti-anginal agent but has modest negative inotropic effects that make it unsuitable for treatment of angina in heart failure patients. Unfortunately, there have been no comparative outcome studies between diltiazem and verapamil.

Dihydropyridines – Long-acting nifedipine is a powerful arterial vasodilator used as an anti-anginal agent particularly in coronary artery disease patients with hypertension, often added to a beta-blocker [67]. Amlodipine, another member of this group, has a long half-life and has been shown to be an effective anti-anginal [68] and antihypertensive agent given as a single daily dose of 5 or 10 mg. In a large study with non-hypertensive coronary disease patients, amlodipine was shown to reduce cardiovascular events over a 24-month follow up [69]. Side-effects include ankle oedema and hypotension.

Nicorandil

Nicorandil acts as both a nitric oxide donor and a sarcolemmal K+–adenosine triphosphate (K-ATP)-dependant channel opener, causing K+ efflux and subsequent hyperpolarisation and inhibition of L-type Ca2+ channels, leading to systemic and coronary vasodilatation. The beneficial effects of nicorandil monotherapy are similar to those of metoprolol, amlodipine, diltiazem and nitrates [70–73].

In the IONA (Impact Of Nicorandil in Angina) study, a reduced rate of fatal and non-fatal myocardial infarction and reduced admission for cardiac chest pain were seen in patients taking nicorandil in addition to other standard anti-anginal therapies [74]. The cardio-protective properties of nicorandil might be due to ischaemic preconditioning mediated by activation of mitochondrial K-ATP channels [75]. Nicorandil also appears to have a protective effect on endothelial function [76–78].

Several theories have been proposed to explain potential cardioprotective properties of nicorandil. One hypothesis is that K-ATP channel opening mimics actions of endogenous adenosine release, thereby shortening myocardial cell action potentials, and reducing Ca2+ overload and cellular energy demands [75, 79].

Nicorandil is rapidly and almost completely absorbed via the gastrointestinal tract, reaching maximal plasma concentration after 30–60 min, and steady-state levels following 4–5 days of standard therapy. Gastrointestinal absorption is delayed, but not decreased by food. Its half-life is roughly 52 min and nicorandil does not undergo first-pass metabolism. Nicorandil circulates largely unbound to albumin or other plasma proteins. Its anti-anginal effects last approximately 12 h, necessitating twice-daily dosage. Pharmacokinetic properties are not significantly affected by age, chronic liver and/or renal disease. Metformin might antagonise the effects of nicorandil by closing K-ATP channels [80].

A usual starting dose of nicorandil is 10 mg twice daily, or 5 mg for patients susceptible to headache. The therapeutic dose is typically 10–20 mg twice daily, and maximum dose 30 mg twice daily. Unlike nitrates, tolerance to nicorandil does not tend to occur, probably due to its dual mode of action [81, 82]. However, an attenuated response during exercise testing was reported in one study, after 2 weeks of sustained therapy. Nicorandil does not cause rebound angina [83]. The lowest effective dose is recommended to avoid potential side effects. Common side effects of nicorandil are headaches, dizziness, nausea, vomiting and flushing. The use of phosphodiesterase-5 inhibitors and nitrates should be avoided by those taking nicorandil because of the risk of profound systemic hypotension. Physicians should be alerted as to the possible occurrence of mouth and gut ulceration with the use of nicorandil. The development of this undesirable effect requires the immediate discuntinuation of nicorandil.

Ivabradine

Ivabradine is a selective heart-rate–lowering (physiological) agent that inhibits the *If* current in the pacemaker cells in the sino-atrial node. It is approved for treatment of heart failure with a goal of preventing hospitalization in patients who have an increased heart rate despite adequate beta-blocker therapy. It has also been approved for symptomatic therapy of angina and reported to be as effective as atenolol [84, 85] and amlodipine [86] in improving exercise duration in patients with chronic stable angina who are not receiving background therapy [54] and in combination with atenolol [85].

This is not surprising as myocardial ischaemia is mainly related to increased myocardial oxygen consumption that cannot be matched by an increase in coronary blood flow, due to the presence of coronary stenoses. Myocardial perfusion occurs predominantly during diastole and there is an inverse relationship between perfusion time and heart rate, with subendocardial perfusion being particularly sensitive to an increased heart rate [84, 85].

Increased heart rate commonly precedes effort-induced ischemia and is also an independent risk factor for serious cardiovascular events, particularly in the presence of left ventricular systolic dysfunction [87, 88]. In patients with a previous myocardial infarction, mortality was reported to increase in subjects with baseline heart rates >60 bpm [89]. Therefore, reducing heart rate is a rational strategy to reduce myocardial ischaemia and to prevent cardiac events, particularly in patients with heart failure.

Both beta-blockers and non-dihydropyridine calcium channel blockers reduce heart rate and improve angina. In everyday clinical practice, however, many patients remain symptomatic on beta blockers or calcium channel blockers and therefore the addition of ivabradine, which selectively reduces heart rate, represents an important therapeutic option for the management of patients with stable angina.

Used as monotherapy, ivabradine has been shown to have beneficial effects similar to those of beta-blockers and calcium channel blockers in exercise induced angina [85].

The ASSOCIATE trial, in 889 patients with chronic stable angina, showed that the addition of ivabradine to standard atenolol therapy resulted in improvements in all exercise capacity parameters [85] (Fig. 6.3).

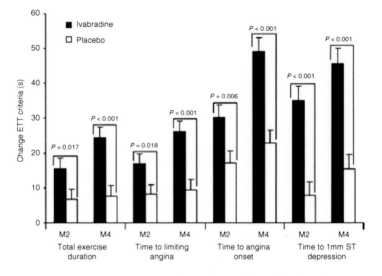

FIGURE 6.3 The ASSOCIATE trial, in 889 patients with chronic stable angina, showed that the addition of ivabradine to standard atenolol therapy resulted in improvements in all exercise capacity parameters (Ref. [85], with permission). The association of ivabradine and atenolol improves exercise stress testing results in patients with stable angina

Moreover, recent data from ADDITIONS (PrActical Daily efficacy anD safety of Procoralan(®) In combinaTION with betablockerS) study, involving 2330 patients with stable angina who were treated with a flexible dose of ivabradine twice daily in addition to beta-blockers for 4 months [90], showed that combined treatment with ivabradine and metoprolol reduced heart rate, the frequency of angina attacks and nitrate consumption, leading to improved QoL. The combination of ivabradine and metoprolol was safe and well tolerated by patients and may represent a useful therapeutic strategy. This combined formulation – ivabradine and metoprolol (Implicor) – is now available in clinical practice.

Effects of Ivabradine Over and Above Decreased Oxygen Demand due to Heart Rate Reduction The main postulated anti-anginal mechanism of ivabradine is the reduction of myocardial oxygen consumption via a heart-rate reducing effect. Experimental and clinical studies, however, have shown that ivabradine may exert its anti-ischaemic effects through other mechanisms. Camici et al. recently reviewed the topic in a scholarly paper [91]. Three main mechanisms were reviewed by Camici et al. [91], i.e. effects on diastolic time, improved endothelial function, and increased coronary flow reserve.

Effects on Diastolic Time and Subendocardial Perfusion As coronary blood flow occurs mostly during diastole, diastolic time is of major importance to ensure adequate blood supply to the myocardium. Moreover, the subendocardium is particularly susceptible to ischaemia and therefore increasing diastolic duration has a beneficial action. Beta-blockers reduce heart rate, which decreases myocardial oxygen demand and they also increase diastolic time. The effects of both ivabradine and the beta-blocker atenolol on diastolic duration, and resulting coronary blood flow changes, were compared in dogs. Ivabradine increased diastolic duration at rest and during exercise to a greater extent than atenolol, and a larger increase in coronary blood flow was observed, despite a similar reduction in heart rate with both agents [92].

Similar findings were reported by Dillinger et al. in patients with coronary artery disease receiving treatment with beta-blockers [93] (Fig. 6.4).

Effect on Coronary Blood Flow Reserve Coronary flow velocity reserve (CFVR) is a prognostic marker in patients with stable coronary artery disease. In a small study of 59 patients, Tagliamonte et al. [94] compared the effects of bisoprolol and ivabradine on CFVR in patients with stable coronary artery disease. Patients in sinus rhythm with stable coronary artery disease were enrolled in a prospective, randomized, double-blind trial. Transthoracic Doppler-derived CFVR was assessed in the left anterior descending coronary artery, and was calculated as the ratio of hyperaemic to baseline diastolic coronary flow velocity (CFV). Hyperaemic CFV was obtained with dipyridamole administration using standard protocols. After CFVR assessment, patients were randomized to ivabradine or bisoprolol and entered an up-titration phase, and

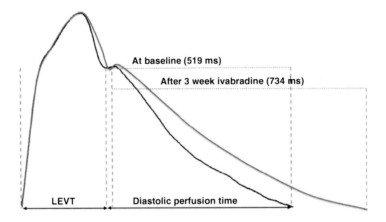

FIGURE 6.4 Schematic representation of the prolongation of diastolic tine with ivabradine in patients with stable coronary artery disease during a single heart beat at rest. *LVET* indicates left ventricular ejection time (From Ref. [93] with permission)

CFVR was assessed again 1 month after the end of the up-titration phase. Fifty-nine patients (38 male, 21 female; mean age 69 ± 9 years) were enrolled. Transthoracic Doppler-derived assessment of CFV and CFVR was successfully performed in all patients. Baseline characteristics were similar in the bisoprolol and ivabradine groups.

At baseline, rest and hyperemic peak CFV as well as CFVR was not significantly different in the ivabradine and bisoprolol groups. With treatment, resting peak CFV significantly decreased in both the ivabradine and bisoprolol groups, but there was no significant difference between the groups (ivabradine group 20.7 ± 4.6 vs. 22.8 ± 5.2, $p < 0.001$; bisoprolol group 20.1 ± 4.1 vs. 22.1 ± 4.3, $p < 0.001$). However, hyperemic peak CFV significantly increased in both groups, but to a greater extent in patients treated with ivabradine (ivabradine: 70.7 ± 9.4 vs. 58.8 ± 9.2, $p < 0.001$; bisoprolol: 65 ± 8.3 vs. 58.7 ± 8.2, $p < 0.001$). Accordingly, CFVR significantly increased in both groups (ivabradine 3.52 ± 0.64 vs. 2.67 ± 0.55, $p < 0.001$; bisoprolol 3.35 ± 0.70 vs. 2.72 ± 0.55,

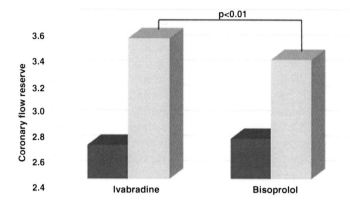

FIGURE 6.5 Ivabradine improves hyperaemic peak CFV and CFVR to a greater extent than bisoprolol in patients with stable coronary artery disease, despite a similar decrease in heart rate (From Ref. [94] with permission)

$p < 0.001$), but it was significantly higher in the ivabradine group, despite a similar decrease in heart rate (63 ± 7 vs. 61 ± 6; P not significant). Thus ivabradine improves hyperemic peak CFV and CFVR to a greater extent than bisoprolol in patients with stable coronary artery disease, despite a similar decrease in heart rate (Fig. 6.5).

These data demonstrate that the benefits from ivabradine therapy go beyond heart rate reduction. This could be due to a different mechanism, such as improved diastolic perfusion time, isovolumetric ventricular relaxation, reduced end-diastolic pressure, and effects on collaterals. Skalidis et al. [95] showed that ivabradine treatment significantly improves hyperaemic coronary flow velocity and CFR in patients with stable coronary artery disease. These effects persisted even after correcting for heart rate, indicating improved coronary microvascular function.

Effects on collateral blood flow. A small study by Gloekler et al. [96] assessed the effect of heart rate reduction by ivabradine on coronary collateral function in patients with chronic stable coronary artery disease. This was a prospective randomised placebo-controlled single centre trial in a university hospital setting. Forty-six patients with chronic stable angina received placebo (n = 23) or ivabradine (n = 23) for 6 months. The main outcome measure was collateral flow index (CFI) as obtained during a 1 min coronary artery balloon occlusion at study inclusion (baseline) and at 6-months of follow-up. CFI is the ratio between simultaneously recorded mean coronary occlusive pressure divided by mean aortic pressure, both subtracted by mean central venous pressure. In the placebo group, CFI decreased from 0.140 ± 0.097 at baseline to 0.109 ± 0.067 at follow-up (p = 0.12); it increased from 0.107 ± 0.077 at baseline to 0.152 ± 0.090 at follow-up in the ivabradine group (p = 0.0461). These results suggest that heart rate reduction by ivabradine has a beneficial effect on coronary collateral function in patients with chronic stable angina. Ivabradine may also have a preventative effect on the deterioration of endothelial function. In dyslipidaemic mice models of oxidative stress and endothelial dysfunction, treatment with ivabradine prevented the deterioration of endothelium-dependent vasodilation in renal and cerebral arteries. The beta blocker metoprolol, however, did not have such a protective effect despite producing a similar reduction of heart rate [98]. In another experimental model, ivabradine reduced atherosclerotic plaque formation in the aortic root and the ascending aorta of mice [99]. Recent studies in patients with stable coronary artery disease suggest a similarly positive effect of ivabradine on endothelial function [87].

In contrast to beta-blockers and non-dihydropiridine-calcium channel blockers, ivabradine-induced heart rate reduction does not affect myocardial contractility, atrioventricular conduction or ventricular repolarisation [92]. Ivabradine can be used in association with beta blockers or instead of beta blockers, when these are contraindicated. Of importance in clinical practice, proton pump inhibitors, sildenafil, statins, dihydropyridine calcium-channel blockers, digoxin and warfarin do not appear to have any significant effect on the pharmacokinetics and pharmacodynamics of ivabradine.

Ivabradine and Clinical Outcomes

The International multi-centre randomised double-blind placebo controlled trial BEAUTIFUL (morBidity-mortality EvAlUaTion of the If inhibitor ivabradine in patients with coronary disease and left-ventricULar dysfunction), assessed whether reduction of heart rate with ivabradine (5–7.5 mg BD) in patients with stable coronary artery disease and LVEF <40 % on established standard therapy could reduce mortality and morbidity [100]. The primary endpoint was the composite of cardiovascular death, admission to hospital for acute myocardial infarction, and admission to hospital for new-onset or worsening heart failure.

All randomised patients were followed up for 12 months. Of 12,473 patients screened to enter the study, 10,917 eligible patients were randomised to receive either placebo (5438 patients) or ivabradine (5479 patients). Mean HR was 71.6 bpm with 87 % of patients receiving beta blockers at randomisation. Ivabradine was well tolerated and significantly reduced heart rate by 6 bpm at 12 months compared to placebo. No significant improvement in the primary endpoint was observed when ivabradine and placebo treated patients were compared (15.4 % v 15.3 %, hazard ratio 1.00, 95 % CI 0.91–1.1, p = 0.94).

Two major post-hoc analyses of the BEAUTIFUL trial have been reported [97]. The first comprised an analysis of patients randomised to the placebo arm of the study to investigate the relationship between resting HR and clinical outcomes [88] and the second examined the effects of ivabradine therapy in those patients with limiting angina. In the latter, an analysis of 1507 patients in the BEAUTIFUL trial population with limiting angina [97], ivabradine treatment was associated with a significant reduction in the primary endpoint (hazard ratio 0.76, 95 % CI 0.58–1.00, p = 0.05)

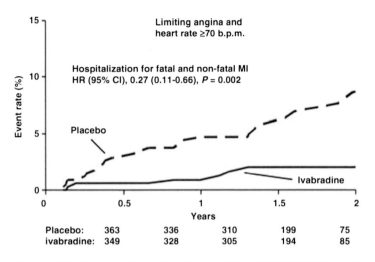

FIGURE 6.6 Results of a subanalysis of the BEAUTIFUL study (From Ref. [97] with permission)

and a significant reduction in hospitalisation for MI (hazard ratio 0.58, 95 % CI 0.37–0.92, p = 0.021) (Fig. 6.6).

The SIGNIFY (Study Assessing the Morbidity–Mortality Benefits of the If Inhibitor Ivabradine) trial recruited 19,102 patients in 51 countries [101]. Patients were randomised to receive ivabradine at an initial dose of 7.5 mg BD (except patients >75 years old who received a dose of 5 mg BD) or placebo. The mean study-drug dose was 8.2 ± 1.7 mg BD in the ivabradine treatment arm. At 3 months, mean HR in the ivabradine treated group was 60.7 ± 9.0 bpm compared with 70.6 ± 10.1 bpm in the placebo arm, with this difference in HR being maintained for the duration of the study. Compliance with study medication was high. Change in beta-blocker dose was infrequent in both study arms. Intention to treat analysis failed to demonstrate any difference in the primary composite endpoint (hazard ratio 1.08; 95 % CI 0.96–1.20, p = 0.20).

All-cause death, cardiovascular death and sudden death were not significantly different in the two groups. Anginal symptoms significantly improved in patients randomised to ivabradine (p = 0.01). Ivabradine was associated with an increase in the incidence of the primary end point among patients with activity-limiting angina (p = 0.02 for interaction).The rates of death and nonfatal myocardial infarction were higher among patients who received ivabradine than among those who received placebo (7.6 % vs. 6.5 %, p = 0.02) [101]. These unexpected findings were followed by intense data analysis and scrutiny to confirm the safety of ivabradine. After this phase was concluded, the European Medicines Agency (EMA) concluded that the risk–benefit ratio to reduce the symptoms of angina remained positive, provided that ivabradine is administered at the usual dosage of 5 mg b.i.d. and uptitrated to 7.5 mg b.i.d., and not given in combination with verapamil or diltiazem and is not used in patients with angina in sinus rhythm who remain symptomatic and with a heart rate ≥70 b.p.m. despite antianginal treatment.

There was no interaction between the use of ivabradine and adverse events in other pre-specified sub-groups, defined according to age, beta blocker use at randomisation, gender, baseline HR, history of diabetes mellitus, previous MI, or previous coronary revascularisation. Ivabradine treatment, compared with placebo, was associated with significantly increased rates of symptomatic (7.9 % v 1.2 %, p < 0.001) and asymptomatic (11.0 % v 1.3 %, p < 0.001) bradycardia, atrial fibrillation (5.3 % v 3.8 %, p < 0.001) and phosphenes (5.4 % v 0.5 %, p < 0.001). However, further analysis of these data demonstrated that both in the whole study as well as in the angina patient subset, neither bradycardia nor atrial fibrillation – in ivabradine-treated patients – affected clinical outcomes compared with placebo [102].

There was an absolute 2.2 % increase in serious adverse events in the ivabradine treated group (p = 0.001). The results of this study indicate that ivabradine significantly improves angina in patients with SCAD but do not support the hypothesis that this drug improves prognosis in patients with SCAD. Ivabradine remains indicated as a second line drug for treatment of symptomatic angina in NICE [15] and ESC guidelines [14].

Drugs That Improve Myocardial Ischaemia Without Affecting Heart Rate or Cardiovascular Haemodynamics

Trimetazidine

Cardiac Energy Metabolism and Myocardial Ischemia

The healthy heart derives most of its energy from the free fatty acid (FFA) metabolic pathway which accounts for approximately two thirds of energy production (adenosine triphosphate – ATP). Another major source of energy results from glucose oxidation and lactate. The healthy heart modulates substrate utilization according to substrate availability, general nutritional status, and myocardial metabolic demand. During mild to moderate myocardial ischemia the myocyte accelerates FFA uptake to generate sufficient ATP to maintain ionic gradients and calcium homeostasis. FFA oxidation requires a greater amount of oxygen than glucose oxidation. During prolonged and severe ischemia the myocardium continues to derive most of its energy from beta-oxidation, despite a high rate of lactate production. High rates of FFA oxidation inhibit glucose oxidation due to competitive interaction (the Randle phenomenon). During ischaemia, FFA oxidation requires more oxygen than glucose metabolism and results in less ATP production and increased oxidative stress. These metabolic changes have profound effects on cell homeostasis ultimately leading to myocyte cell death [103–105].

Trimetazidine's metabolic actions have been shown to have anti-ischaemic properties (Fig. 6.7).

Anti-ischaemic Effects of Trimetazidine

Trimetazidine partially inhibits myocardial FFA oxidation (Fig. 6.7). Kantor et al. showed that trimetazidine specifically inhibits the enzyme acetyl-CoA C-acyltransferase (3-KAT). 3-KAT catalyzes FFA beta-oxidation, with long-chain

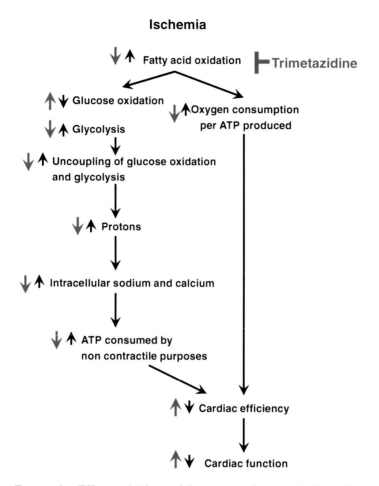

FIGURE 6.7 Effects of trimetazidine on cardiac metabolism. The alteration in fatty acid oxidation during cardiac ischemia is accompanied by an increase in glycolysis and a decrease in glucose oxidation, with deleterious consequences for cardiac homeostasis and efficiency (*black arrows*). The inhibition of fatty acid oxidation with trimetazidine restores the coupling of glycolysis to glucose oxidation, which in turn increases stores of ATP and restores cell function (*red arrows*) (Modified after Fillmore et al. [106]. © 2014, The British Pharmacological Society)

3-ketoacyl-CoA as a substrate for the generation of acetyl-CoA [107].

A preconditioning effect was suggested as an additional reason for some of the beneficial effects of this agent [108, 109]. The antianginal effects of trimetazidine, when given alone or in combination with conventional antianginal drugs, have been shown in many relatively small studies [110].

In the TRIMPOL II trial, a randomized double-blind placebo-controlled multicenter study of 426 patients with stable angina, the combined actions of trimetazidine (20 mg t.d.s) and metoprolol improved total exercise duration, time to ST segment depression, mean nitrate consumption, and angina frequency compared to the use of metoprolol and placebo [111] (Fig. 6.8).

The antianginal efficacy and tolerability of trimetazidine when used in combination with beta-blockers or long-acting nitrates was assessed in the Trimetazidine in Angina Combination Therapy (TACT) study [112].

This randomized, placebo-controlled study enrolled 177 patients with stable angina symptoms that were not controlled by nitrates or beta-blockers. After 12 weeks of treatment, exercise duration, time to 1-mm ST segment depression and time to angina significantly increased in the trimetazidine group. These results are in agreement with findings in a study by Michaelides et al. [113] which showed that the addition of trimetazidine significantly decreased the number of angina attacks (63 % reduction). This was a twofold reduction compared to that achieved by isosorbide dinitrate [52]. Similar results were reported by the VASCO-angina study, a randomized double-blind placebo-controlled trial, which assessed the anti-anginal efficacy and safety of standard and high dose of modified-release trimetazidine in symptomatic and asymptomatic patients with chronic ischemic heart disease [114]. Results of a recent meta-analysis also support the antianginal effect of trimetazidine in patients with stable ischemic heart disease [115].

Interestingly and of practical significance, the beneficial effects of trimetazidine on angina take place without actions on the heart rate or the blood pressure. Of interest, albeit beyond the scope of this chapter, trimetazidine has been shown to improve clinical parameters and survival in patients

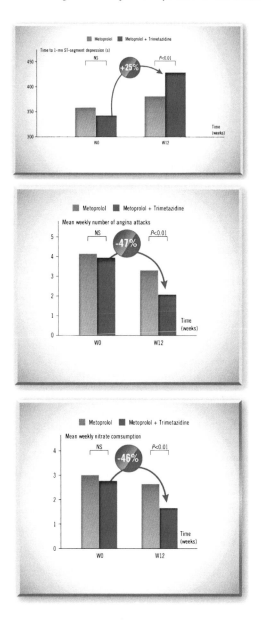

FIGURE 6.8 Results of the TRIMPOL study (From Ref. [111] with permission)

with chronic heart failure. The agent is particularly effective in patients with ischaemic cardiomyopathy. Furthermore, in animal models of ischemia-reperfusion injury, trimetazidine has been shown to have cardioprotective effects, and this finding is of relevance for patients with stable angina with recurrent episodes of prolonged myocardial ischemia. Of interest, a recent study investigated the effect of trimetazidine on the incidence of stent restenosis and major adverse cardiac and cerebrovascular events (MACCEs) in patients undergoing PCI [116]. A total of 786 patients were randomized, after implantation of a drug-eluting stent, to receive trimetazidine (60 mg daily) on top of standard treatment for at least 30 days or standard treatment only. At 1-year follow-up, patients in the trimetazidine group had a significantly lower incidence of stent restenosis and MACCEs compared with those who received standard treatment only (control group). Interestingly, in an animal model of diabetes, trimetazidine decreased the proliferation of vascular smooth muscle cells and promoted re endothelialization after injury of the carotid artery [117].

Overall, these findings suggest that beyond its antianginal effect, trimetazidine may improve prognosis in patients undergoing revascularization procedures. This hypothesis is currently being tested in the ATPCI (The efficacy and safety of Trimetazidine in Patients with angina pectoris treated by percutaneous Coronary Intervention) study, a large morbidity-mortality trial in 5800 angina patients with a post-PCI follow-up of 2–4 years.

At present, the European guidelines give a class IIb recommendation for the use of trimetazidine in patients with chronic stable angina patients [14].

Perhexiline

Perhexiline is a carnitine palmitoyl transferase –1 (CPT-1) inhibitor with some CPT-2 inhibitory action that has been shown to improve angina pectoris [118] and myocardial efficiency [119]. Inhibition of CPT-1/CPT-2 by perhexiline increases myocardial oxygen utilization efficiency by at least

13 %. However, following perhexiline administration, cardiac efficiency increases by approximately 30 %, therefore suggesting additional mechanisms of action [120].

However, interest in the long term administration of perhexiline has been reduced due to serious hepatotoxicity and neuropathy associated with the use of this agent. The drug requires regular monitoring of plasma levels and makes hepatic or renal dysfunction a relative contraindication for the use of perhexiline [121].

Ranolazine

Ranolazine is a racemic mixture that consists of a 1:1 ratio of (R) and (S) enantiomers at the secondary alcohol that originates from the secondary carbon of the epoxide ring in guaiacol glycidyl ether (GGE/Ran 3). Ranolazine is a piperazine derivative that is thought to exert its anti-anginal effect by inhibiting ischaemic-induced late inward $Na+$ currents, preventing $Ca2+$ overload and reducing diastolic wall tension and extrinsic coronary artery compression [122, 123].

Ranolazine might also improve endothelial-mediated coronary vasodilatation [124]. Ranolazine was approved for clinical use in the USA in 2006, as add-on therapy for the treatment of chronic angina, and received a first-line indication in November 2008. The maximum approved dose in the USA is 1 g twice daily. In Europe, ranolazine (prolonged-release tablets) was approved by the European Medicines Agency in July 2008, with a recommended initial dose of 375 mg twice daily that can be further titrated to the recommended maximum dose of 750 mg twice daily. Ranolazine was originally thought to act by affecting cardiac metabolism, i.e. inhibiting beta oxidation; however, the concentration of ranolazine required to inhibit myocardial fatty-acid oxidation is much higher than the therapeutic levels used to treat angina [122]. Ranolazine does not cause significant haemodynamic changes, except for an extremely small reduction (less than 2 beats per minute on average) in heart rate and less than 3 mmHg decrease in systolic blood pressure [80].

The clinical efficacy of ranolazine in chronic stable angina, as monotherapy and in combination with other anti-anginal drugs, has been shown in MARISA (Monotherapy Assessment of Ranolazine in Stable Angina). The MARISA study assessed the tolerability of three doses of ranolazine sustained-release (500, 1000 and 1500 mg) compared to placebo and their effects on treadmill exercise performance in a double-blind, randomised, placebo-controlled, single cross-over study. The study showed a statistically significant improvement in exercise duration compared to placebo for all three doses of ranolazine from 24 s at 500 mg bid. to 46 s at 1500 mg bid. with a clear dose–response pattern. However, given the significant incidence of adverse events in patients receiving the 1500 mg bid dose, the study led to a maximum recommended dosage of 1000 mg bid [125].

CARISA (Combination Assessment of Ranolazine in Stable Angina) [126]

In the CARISA study 823 patients with chronic stable angina were randomised to either ranolazine 750 mg bid. (n = 279), ranolazine 1 g bid or placebo as add-on treatment to atenolol 50 mg od, amlodipine 5 mg od, or diltiazem 180 mg od. Twenty-three percent of the patients were diabetics and 29 % had heart failure, over 60 % were hypertensives and 58 % had suffered a previous myocardial infarction. The primary efficacy end point was the change from baseline in exercise duration at trough after 12 weeks on study drugs. The mean increases in exercise duration at trough were statistically significantly greater for patients treated with either dose of ranolazine SR than with placebo. A significant improvement in the occurrence of anginal episodes and rediction in the use of sublingual nitrates was also observed with ranolazine.

ERICA (Efficacy of Ranolazine in Chronic Angina) Trials [127]

The randomized placebo controlled parallel study ERICA assessed the effect of ranolazine, in patients with coronary artery disease and chronic stable angina with persistent symptoms despite treatment (amlodipine 10 mg daily). Patients allocated to ranolazine showed a significantly lower weekly episodes of angina compared with patients receiving placebo. The effect on angina was mirrored by a significant reduction in the average weekly rate of NTG consumption.

The TERISA study (Type 2 Diabetes Evaluation of Ranolazine in Subjects With Chronic Stable Angina) assessed, in a parallel 8 week double-blind placebo controlled study, the effect of rano-lazine on the occurrence of angina and the use of sublingual nitroglycerin in 949 diabetic patients with coronary artery disease and chronic stable angina treated with up to 2 anti-anginal agents. Ranolazine significantly reduced both angina episodes, compared to placebo (3.8 vs. 4.3 episodes, p=0.008), and the use of sublingual nitrates (1.7 vs. 2.1, p=0.003) [128].

The recent RIVER-PCI study randomized 2389 patients with a history of chronic stable angina who have had incomplete coronary revascularization to receive ranolazine or placebo. After PCI, the Seattle Angina Questionnaire angina frequency score did not differ between groups. However, a significant improvement in angina frequency was observed with ranolazine at 6 months in patients with diabetes and in those with more severe angina, suggesting a beneficial effect of ranolazine in patients with more myocardial ischaemia [129].

In the MERLIN-TIMI 36 (Metabolic Efficiency with Ranolazine for Less Ischemia in Non-ST-elevation acute coronary syndromes) trial no reduction in cardiovascular death, acute myocardial infarction or recurrent ischaemia were seen with ranolazine. A significantly lower incidence of arrhythmias, including ventricular tachycardia, was detected in patients treated with ranolazine compared to patients receiving placebo [130].

Common side effects of ranolazine are: dizziness, nausea, constipation, abdominal pain and headaches. Ranolazine may cause dose-dependent prolongation of the QT-interval. Contraindications to the use of ranolazine are prolonged QT-interval and co-administration with other QT-prolonging drugs, a previous history of ventricular tachycardia, and moderate to severe renal impairment or severe hepatic failure. Co-administration or ranolazine with of Class Ia (such as quinidine) or Class III (such as dofetilide and sotalol) antiar-rhythmics is contraindicated. Ranolazine is metabolised in the liver, CYP3A4, and to a lesser extent, by CYP2D6 enzymes, consequently there is a potential for drug interactions. Ranolazine is also a weak inhibitor of cytochrome p450 enzymes and therefore doses of P-glycoprotein substrates (e.g. simvasatin and digoxin) might need to be reduced in people taking ranolazine [80].

Other Agents

Allopurinol, a xanthine oxidase inhibitor that is used to prevent gout, has also been proposed as an antianginal metabolic agent [131]. Potential mechanisms include decreased demand for myocardial oxygen, improved vascular endothelial function and reduced oxidative stress [132]. In a study involving 65 patients with chronic angina, the time to ischemia with an exercise ECG stress test was longer among persons who received high-dose allopurinol than among those who received placebo [131]. Because of limited clinical data, U.S. guidelines do not recommend allopurinol for the treatment of angina [16] but it is recommended in the European guidelines [14].

Molsidomine. This direct NO donor has anti-ischaemic effects similar to those of isosorbide dinitrate [133]. The long-acting once-daily 16 mg formulation is as effective as 8 mg twice daily [133].

Revascularisation Versus Medical Therapy

Randomised trials involving patients who were eligible for either medical therapy or revascularisation have shown that PCI is effective in reducing symptoms in patients with chronic angina [134, 135].

PCI does not, however, result in a lower risk of death or myocardial infarction compared with optimal medical therapy [136]. These observations suggest that optimal medical therapy is a sensible initial strategic option in most cases. The decision

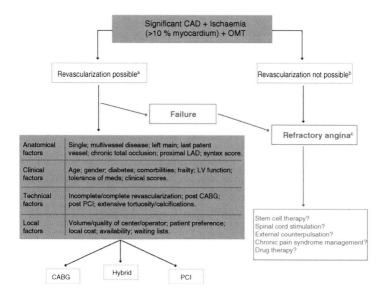

FIGURE 6.9 The decision to proceed to myocardial revascularization should be based on the presence of flow limiting obstructive coronary artery stenosis, the degree of ischaemia and the expected benefit of the intervention regarding prognosis and/or symptoms (From Ref. [14] with permission)

to proceed to myocardial revascularization should be based on the presence of flow limiting obstructive coronary artery stenosis, the degree of ischaemia and the expected benefit of the intervention regarding prognosis and/or symptoms (Fig. 6.9). Clinical, anatomical, technical and environmental factors need to be considered to estimate the potential benefit of revascularization. The measurement of fractional flow reserve, a hemodynamic assessment of the severity of a lesion by measurement of the pressure difference across a lesion in a patient with drug-induced hyperaemia, is useful in defining the clinical significance of borderline lesions [134]. In randomized trials using fractional flow reserve measurements, clinical outcomes were better when only lesions with a fractional flow reserve of 0.80 or less were treated with PCI than when treatment was based on visual assessment of stenosis severity [137, 138].

A meta-analysis of several randomized trials suggested that routine use of fractional flow reserve during diagnostic angiography could reduce the need for revascularization (predominantly PCI) by 50 %, with a relative reduction of 20 % in rates of death, myocardial infarction, and subsequent revascularization procedures [137].

The decision to revascularise with PCI or coronary-artery by-pass grafting, or to continue medical therapy, should ideally involve a heart-team approach with input from the interventional team and the management physician, as recommended by American and European guidelines (Fig. 6.9). The decision should take into account clinical risk factors, characteristics of the lesion, hemodynamic factors, and should be informed by the use of validated clinical and angiographic risk scores [134]. In this regard, for a given patient, consensus among the members of the management team is of paramount importance. Revascularization should be considered for patients who have ongoing angina despite adequate medical therapy; this group includes as many as 50 % of patients with chronic angina [134]. When feasible technically in patients with an acceptable level of risk and good life expectancy, revascularisation is indicated in those with chronic angina refractory to optimal medical therapy. Revascularisation can also be considered first-line treatment in patients with significant left main stenosis. Bypass surgery in patients with 50 % or greater left main lumen diameter reduction is a recommended option, given the striking differences in survival noted in the Veterans Administration Cooperative Study in a subgroup of 113 patients [139, 140], and confirmed in a subsequent meta-analysis [141] as well as studies from the CASS registry [142, 143].

References

1. Ohman EM. Clinical practice. Chronic stable angina. N Engl J Med. 2016;374:1167–76.
2. Mozaffarian D, Benjamin EJ, Go AS, Arnett DK, Blaha MJ, Cushman M, de Ferranti S, Després J-P, Fullerton HJ, Howard

VJ, Huffman MD, Judd SE, Kissela BM, Lackland DT, Lichtman JH, Lisabeth LD, Liu S, Mackey RH, Matchar DB, McGuire DK, Mohler ER, Moy CS, Muntner P, Mussolino ME, Nasir K, Neumar RW, Nichol G, Palaniappan L, Pandey DK, Reeves MJ, et al. Heart disease and stroke statistics – 2015 update: a report from the American Heart Association. Circulation. 2015;131: e29–322.

3. Jones M, Rait G, Falconer J, Feder G. Systematic review: prognosis of angina in primary care. Fam Pract. 2006;23:520–8.

4. Henry TD, Satran D, Hodges JS, Johnson RK, Poulose AK, Campbell AR, Garberich RF, Bart BA, Olson RE, Boisjolie CR, Harvey KL, Arndt TL, Traverse JH. Long-term survival in patients with refractory angina. Eur Heart J. 2013;34:2683–8.

5. Daly CA, De Stavola B, Sendon JLL, Tavazzi L, Boersma E, Clemens F, Danchin N, Delahaye F, Gitt A, Julian D, Mulcahy D, Ruzyllo W, Thygesen K, Verheugt F, Fox KM, Euro Heart Survey Investigators. Predicting prognosis in stable angina – results from the Euro heart survey of stable angina: prospective observational study. BMJ. 2006;332:262–7.

6. Bhatt DL, Eagle KA, Ohman EM, Hirsch AT, Goto S, Mahoney EM, Wilson PWF, Alberts MJ, D'Agostino R, Liau C-S, Mas J-L, Röther J, Smith SC, Salette G, Contant CF, Massaro JM, Steg PG, REACH Registry Investigators. Comparative determinants of 4-year cardiovascular event rates in stable outpatients at risk of or with atherothrombosis. JAMA. 2010;304:1350–7.

7. Povsic TJ, Broderick S, Anstrom KJ, Shaw LK, Ohman EM, Eisenstein EL, Smith PK, Alexander JH. Predictors of long-term clinical endpoints in patients with refractory angina. J Am Heart Assoc. 2015;4:1–12.

8. Kaski JC, Rosano GM, Collins P, Nihoyannopoulos P, Maseri A, Poole-Wilson PA. Cardiac syndrome X: clinical characteristics and left ventricular function. Long-term follow-up study. J Am Coll Cardiol. 1995;25:807–14.

9. Kaski JC. Pathophysiology and management of patients with chest pain and normal coronary arteriograms (cardiac syndrome X). Circulation. 2004;109:568–72.

10. Camici PG, Crea F. Coronary microvascular dysfunction. N Engl J Med. 2007;356:830–40.

11. Murthy VL, Naya M, Taqueti VR, Foster CR, Gaber M, Hainer J, Dorbala S, Blankstein R, Rimoldi O, Camici PG, Di Carli MF. Effects of sex on coronary microvascular dysfunction and cardiac outcomes. Circulation. 2014;129:2518–27.

12. Pepine CJ, Anderson RD, Sharaf BL, Reis SE, Smith KM, Handberg EM, Johnson BD, Sopko G, Bairey Merz CN. Coronary microvascular reactivity to adenosine predicts adverse outcome in women evaluated for suspected ischemia results from the National Heart, Lung and Blood Institute WISE (Women's Ischemia Syndrome Evaluation) study. J Am Coll Cardiol. 2010;55:2825–32.

13. Jespersen L, Hvelplund A, Abildstrøm SZ, Pedersen F, Galatius S, Madsen JK, Jørgensen E, Kelbæk H, Prescott E. Stable angina pectoris with no obstructive coronary artery disease is associated with increased risks of major adverse cardiovascular events. Eur Heart J. 2012;33:734–44.

14. Montalescot G, Sechtem U, Achenbach S, Andreotti F, Arden C, Budaj A, Bugiardini R, Crea F, Cuisset T, Di Mario C, Ferreira JR, Gersh BJ, Gitt AK, Hulot JS, Marx N, Opie LH, Pfisterer M, Prescott E, Ruschitzka F, Sabaté M, Senior R, Taggart DP, Van Der Wall EE, Vrints CJM, Zamorano JL, Baumgartner H, Bax JJ, Bueno H, Dean V, Deaton C, et al. 2013 ESC guidelines on the management of stable coronary artery disease. Eur Heart J. 2013;34:2949–3003.

15. Henderson RA, O'Flynn N. Management of stable angina: summary of NICE guidance. Heart. 2012;98:500–7.

16. Fihn SD, Gardin JM, Abrams J, Berra K, Blankenship JC, Dallas AP, Douglas PS, Foody JM, Gerber TC, Hinderliter AL, King 3rd SB, Kligfield PD, Krumholz HM, Kwong RYK, Lim MJ, Linderbaum JA, Mack MJ, Munger MA, Prager RL, Sabik JF, Shaw LJ, Sikkema JD, Smith CRJ, Smith SCJ, Spertus JA, Williams SV. 2012 ACCF/AHA/ACP/AATS/PCNA/SCAI/STS guideline for the diagnosis and management of patients with stable ischemic heart disease: a report of the American College of Cardiology Foundation/American Heart Association Task Force on Practice Guidelines, and the. J Am Coll Cardiol. 2012;60:e44–164.

17. Kaski J-C, Arrebola-Moreno A, Dungu J. Treatment strategies for chronic stable angina. Expert Opin Pharmacother. 2011;12: 2833–44.

18. Perk J, De Backer G, Gohlke H, Graham I, Reiner Z, Verschuren M, Albus C, Benlian P, Boysen G, Cifkova R, Deaton C, Ebrahim S, Fisher M, Germano G, Hobbs R, Hoes A, Karadeniz S, Mezzani A, Prescott E, Ryden L, Scherer M, Syvänne M, Scholte op Reimer WJM, Vrints C, Wood D, Zamorano JL, Zannad F, European Association for Cardiovascular Prevention & Rehabilitation (EACPR), ESC Committee for Practice

Guidelines (CPG). European guidelines on cardiovascular disease prevention in clinical practice (version 2012). The Fifth Joint Task Force of the European Society of Cardiology and Other Societies on Cardiovascular Disease Prevention in Clinical Practice (constituted by representatives of nine societies and by invited experts). Eur Heart J. 2012;33:1635–701.

19. Kohler M, Stradling JR. Mechanisms of vascular damage in obstructive sleep apnea. Nat Rev Cardiol. 2010;7:677–85.

20. Filion KB, El Khoury F, Bielinski M, Schiller I, Dendukuri N, Brophy JM. Omega-3 fatty acids in high-risk cardiovascular patients: a meta-analysis of randomized controlled trials. BMC Cardiovasc Disord. 2010;10:24.

21. Mozaffarian D, Wu JHY. Omega-3 fatty acids and cardiovascular disease: effects on risk factors, molecular pathways, and clinical events. J Am Coll Cardiol. 2011;58:2047–67.

22. Kwak SM, Myung S-K, Lee YJ, Seo HG, Korean Meta-analysis Study Group. Efficacy of omega-3 fatty acid supplements (eicosapentaenoic acid and docosahexaenoic acid) in the secondary prevention of cardiovascular disease: a meta-analysis of randomized, double-blind, placebo-controlled trials. Arch Intern Med. 2012;172:686–94.

23. Estruch R, Ros E, Salas-Salvadó J, Covas M-I, Corella D, Arós F, Gómez-Gracia E, Ruiz-Gutiérrez V, Fiol M, Lapetra J, Lamuela-Raventos RM, Serra-Majem L, Pintó X, Basora J, Muñoz MA, Sorlí JV, Martínez JA, Martínez-González MA, PREDIMED Study Investigators. Primary prevention of cardiovascular disease with a Mediterranean diet. N Engl J Med. 2013;368:1279–90.

24. European Association for Cardiovascular Prevention & Rehabilitation; Reiner Z, Catapano AL, Backer G De, Graham I, Taskinen M-R, Wiklund O, Agewall S, Alegria E, Chapman MJ, Durrington P, Erdine S, Halcox J, Hobbs R, Kjekshus J, Filardi PP, Riccardi G, Storey RF, Wood D, ESC Committee for Practice Guidelines (CPG) 2008-2010 and 2010-2012 Committees. ESC/EAS Guidelines for the management of dyslipidaemias: the Task Force for the management of dyslipidaemias of the European Society of Cardiology (ESC) and the European Atherosclerosis Society (EAS). Eur Heart J. 2011;32:1769–818.

25. Pasceri V, Patti G, Nusca A, Pristipino C, Richichi G, Di Sciascio G, ARMYDA Investigators. Randomized trial of atorvastatin for reduction of myocardial damage during coronary intervention: results from the ARMYDA (Atorvastatin for Reduction of MYocardial Damage during Angioplasty) study. Circulation. 2004;110:674–8.

26. Deanfield JE, Sellier P, Thaulow E, Bultas J, Yunis C, Shi H, Buch J, Beckerman B. Potent anti-ischaemic effects of statins in chronic stable angina: incremental benefit beyond lipid lowering? Eur Heart J. 2010;31:2650–9.

27. Stone PH, Lloyd-Jones DM, Kinlay S, Frei B, Carlson W, Rubenstein J, Andrews TC, Johnstone M, Sopko G, Cole H, Orav J, Selwyn AP, Creager MA, Vascular Basis Study Group. Effect of intensive lipid lowering, with or without antioxidant vitamins, compared with moderate lipid lowering on myocardial ischemia in patients with stable coronary artery disease: the Vascular Basis for the Treatment of Myocardial Ischemia Study. Circulation. 2005;111:1747–55.

28. Pitt B, Waters D, Brown WV, van Boven AJ, Schwartz L, Title LM, Eisenberg D, Shurzinske L, McCormick LS. Aggressive lipid-lowering therapy compared with angioplasty in stable coronary artery disease. Atorvastatin versus Revascularization Treatment Investigators. N Engl J Med. 1999;341:70–6.

29. Meyers DG, Neuberger JS, He J. Cardiovascular effect of bans on smoking in public places: a systematic review and meta-analysis. J Am Coll Cardiol. 2009;54:1249–55.

30. Lam TH. Absolute Risk of Tobacco Deaths: One in Two Smokers Will Be Killed by Smoking - Comment on "Smoking and All-Cause Mortality in Older People". Arch Intern Med. 2012;172(11):845–6. doi:10.1001/archinternmed.2012.

31. Critchley J, Capewell S. Smoking cessation for the secondary prevention of coronary heart disease. Cochrane Database Syst Rev. 2003;(1);CD003041.

32. Hubbard R, Lewis S, Smith C, Godfrey C, Smeeth L, Farrington P, Britton J. Use of nicotine replacement therapy and the risk of acute myocardial infarction, stroke, and death. Tob Control. 2005;14:416–21.

33. Ludvig J, Miner B, Eisenberg MJ. Smoking cessation in patients with coronary artery disease. Am Heart J. 2005;149:565–72.

34. Singh S, Loke YK, Spangler JG, Furberg CD. Risk of serious adverse cardiovascular events associated with varenicline: a systematic review and meta-analysis. CMAJ. 2011;183:1359–66.

35. Umpierrez GE, Hellman R, Korytkowski MT, Kosiborod M, Maynard GA, Montori VM, Seley JJ, Van den Berghe G, Endocrine Society. Management of hyperglycemia in hospitalized patients in non-critical care setting: an endocrine society clinical practice guideline. J Clin Endocrinol Metab. 2012;97:16–38.

36. SPRINT Research Group, Wright JT, Williamson JD, Whelton PK, Snyder JK, Sink KM, Rocco MV, Reboussin DM, Rahman M, Oparil S, Lewis CE, Kimmel PL, Johnson KC, Goff DC, Fine LJ, Cutler JA, Cushman WC, Cheung AK, Ambrosius WT. A randomized trial of intensive versus standard blood-pressure control. N Engl J Med. 2015;373:2103–16.

37. Mancia G, Laurent S, Agabiti-Rosei E, Ambrosioni E, Burnier M, Caulfield MJ, Cifkova R, Clément D, Coca A, Dominiczak A, Erdine S, Fagard R, Farsang C, Grassi G, Haller H, Heagerty A, Kjeldsen SE, Kiowski W, Mallion JM, Manolis A, Narkiewicz K, Nilsson P, Olsen MH, Rahn KH, Redon J, Rodicio J, Ruilope L, Schmieder RE, Struijker-Boudier HAJ, van Zwieten PA, et al. Reappraisal of European guidelines on hypertension management: a European Society of Hypertension Task Force document. J Hypertens. 2009;27:2121–58.

38. Mancia G, Fagard R, Narkiewicz K, Redon J, Zanchetti A, Böhm M, Christiaens T, Cifkova R, De Backer G, Dominiczak A, Galderisi M, Grobbee DE, Jaarsma T, Kirchhof P, Kjeldsen SE, Laurent S, Manolis AJ, Nilsson PM, Ruilope LM, Schmieder RE, Sirnes PA, Sleight P, Viigimaa M, Waeber B, Zannad F, Redon J, Dominiczak A, Narkiewicz K, Nilsson PM, Burnier M, et al. 2013 ESH/ESC guidelines for the management of arterial hypertension: the Task Force for the Management of Arterial Hypertension of the European Society of Hypertension (ESH) and of the European Society of Cardiology (ESC). Eur Heart J. 2013;34: 2159–219.

39. Manson JE, Hsia J, Johnson KC, Rossouw JE, Assaf AR, Lasser NL, Trevisan M, Black HR, Heckbert SR, Detrano R, Strickland OL, Wong ND, Crouse JR, Stein E, Cushman M, Women's Health Initiative Investigators. Estrogen plus progestin and the risk of coronary heart disease. N Engl J Med. 2003;349:523–34.

40. Collaborative overview of randomised trials of antiplatelet therapy – I: prevention of death, myocardial infarction, and stroke by prolonged antiplatelet therapy in various categories of patients. Antiplatelet Trialists' Collaboration. BMJ. 1994;308: 81–106.

41. Antithrombotic Trialists' Collaboration. Collaborative meta-analysis of randomised trials of antiplatelet therapy for prevention of death, myocardial infarction, and stroke in high risk patients. BMJ. 2002;324:71–86.

42. Juul-Möller S, Edvardsson N, Jahnmatz B, Rosén A, Sørensen S, Omblus R. Double-blind trial of aspirin in primary prevention of

myocardial infarction in patients with stable chronic angina pectoris. The Swedish Angina Pectoris Aspirin Trial (SAPAT) Group. Lancet. 1992;340:1421–5.

43. Antithrombotic Trialists' (ATT) Collaboration; Baigent C, Blackwell L, Collins R, Emberson J, Godwin J, Peto R, Buring J, Hennekens C, Kearney P, Meade T, Patrono C, Roncaglioni MC, Zanchetti A. Aspirin in the primary and secondary prevention of vascular disease: collaborative meta-analysis of individual participant data from randomised trials. Lancet. 2009;373: 1849–60.

44. CAPRIE Steering Committee. A randomised, blinded, trial of clopidogrel versus aspirin in patients at risk of ischaemic events (CAPRIE). CAPRIE Steering Committee. Lancet. 1996;348: 1329–39.

45. Gurbel PA, Bliden KP, Butler K, Tantry US, Gesheff T, Wei C, Teng R, Antonino MJ, Patil SB, Karunakaran A, Kereiakes DJ, Parris C, Purdy D, Wilson V, Ledley GS, Storey RF. Randomized double-blind assessment of the ONSET and OFFSET of the antiplatelet effects of ticagrelor versus clopidogrel in patients with stable coronary artery disease: the ONSET/OFFSET study. Circulation. 2009;120:2577–85.

46. Jernberg T, Payne CD, Winters KJ, Darstein C, Brandt JT, Jakubowski JA, Naganuma H, Siegbahn A, Wallentin L. Prasugrel achieves greater inhibition of platelet aggregation and a lower rate of non-responders compared with clopidogrel in aspirin-treated patients with stable coronary artery disease. Eur Heart J. 2006;27:1166–73.

47. Wiviott SD, Braunwald E, McCabe CH, Montalescot G, Ruzyllo W, Gottlieb S, Neumann F-J, Ardissino D, De Servi S, Murphy SA, Riesmeyer J, Weerakkody G, Gibson CM, Antman EM, TRITON-TIMI 38 Investigators. Prasugrel versus clopidogrel in patients with acute coronary syndromes. N Engl J Med. 2007;357:2001–15.

48. Cannon CP, Harrington RA, James S, Ardissino D, Becker RC, Emanuelsson H, Husted S, Katus H, Keltai M, Khurmi NS, Kontny F, Lewis BS, Steg PG, Storey RF, Wojdyla D, Wallentin L, PLATelet inhibition and patient Outcomes Investigators. Comparison of ticagrelor with clopidogrel in patients with a planned invasive strategy for acute coronary syndromes (PLATO): a randomised double-blind study. Lancet. 2010;375:283–93.

49. Bhatt DL, Fox KAA, Hacke W, Berger PB, Black HR, Boden WE, Cacoub P, Cohen EA, Creager MA, Easton JD, Flather MD,

Haffner SM, Hamm CW, Hankey GJ, Johnston SC, Mak K-H, Mas J-L, Montalescot G, Pearson TA, Steg PG, Steinhubl SR, Weber MA, Brennan DM, Fabry-Ribaudo L, Booth J, Topol EJ, CHARISMA Investigators. Clopidogrel and aspirin versus aspirin alone for the prevention of atherothrombotic events. N Engl J Med. 2006;354:1706–17.

50. Bhatt DL, Flather MD, Hacke W, Berger PB, Black HR, Boden WE, Cacoub P, Cohen EA, Creager MA, Easton JD, Hamm CW, Hankey GJ, Johnston SC, Mak K-H, Mas J-L, Montalescot G, Pearson TA, Steg PG, Steinhubl SR, Weber MA, Fabry-Ribaudo L, Hu T, Topol EJ, Fox KAA, CHARISMA Investigators. Patients with prior myocardial infarction, stroke, or symptomatic peripheral arterial disease in the CHARISMA trial. J Am Coll Cardiol. 2007;49:1982–8.

51. Fox KM. EURopean trial On reduction of cardiac events with Perindopril in stable coronary Artery disease Investigators. Efficacy of perindopril in reduction of cardiovascular events among patients with stable coronary artery disease: randomised, double-blind, placebo-controlled, multicentre trial (the EUROPA study). Lancet. 2003;362:782–8.

52. Strauss MH, Hall AS. The divergent cardiovascular effects of angiotensin converting enzyme inhibitors and angiotensin receptor blockers on myocardial infarction and death. Prog Cardiovasc Dis. 2016;58:473–82.

53. Bertrand ME, Ferrari R, Remme WJ, Simoons ML, Fox KM. Perindopril and β-blocker for the prevention of cardiac events and mortality in stable coronary artery disease patients: a EUropean trial on Reduction Of cardiac events with Perindopril in stable coronary Artery disease (EUROPA) subanalysis. Am Heart J. 2015;170:1092–8.

54. Husted SE, Ohman EM. Pharmacological and emerging therapies in the treatment of chronic angina. Lancet. 2015;386: 691–701.

55. Thadani U, Fung HL, Darke AC, Parker JO. Oral isosorbide dinitrate in angina pectoris: comparison of duration of action an dose-response relation during acute and sustained therapy. Am J Cardiol. 1982;49:411–9.

56. Parker JO. Eccentric dosing with isosorbide-5-mononitrate in angina pectoris. Am J Cardiol. 1993;72:871–6.

57. Chrysant SG, Glasser SP, Bittar N, Shahidi FE, Danisa K, Ibrahim R, Watts LE, Garutti RJ, Ferraresi R, Casareto R. Efficacy and safety of extended-release isosorbide mononi-

trate for stable effort angina pectoris. Am J Cardiol. 1993;72: 1249–56.
58. Bangalore S, Steg G, Deedwania P, Crowley K, Eagle KA, Goto S, Ohman EM, Cannon CP, Smith SC, Zeymer U, Hoffman EB, Messerli FH, Bhatt DL. REACH Registry Investigators. β-Blocker use and clinical outcomes in stable outpatients with and without coronary artery disease. JAMA. 2012;308:1340–9.
59. Bangalore S, Bhatt DL, Steg PG, Weber MA, Boden WE, Hamm CW, Montalescot G, Hsu A, Fox KAA, Lincoff AM. β-blockers and cardiovascular events in patients with and without myocardial infarction: post hoc analysis from the CHARISMA trial. Circ Cardiovasc Qual Outcomes. 2014;7:872–81.
60. Fox KM, Mulcahy D, Findlay I, Ford I, Dargie HJ. The Total Ischaemic Burden European Trial (TIBET). Effects of atenolol, nifedipine SR and their combination on the exercise test and the total ischaemic burden in 608 patients with stable angina. The TIBET Study Group. Eur Heart J. 1996;17:96–103.
61. Rehnqvist N, Hjemdahl P, Billing E, Björkander I, Eriksson SV, Forslund L, Held C, Näsman P, Wallén NH. Effects of metoprolol vs verapamil in patients with stable angina pectoris. The Angina Prognosis Study in Stockholm (APSIS). Eur Heart J. 1996;17:76–81.
62. Hjalmarson A, Goldstein S, Fagerberg B, Wedel H, Waagstein F, Kjekshus J, Wikstrand J, El Allaf D, Vítovec J, Aldershvile J, Halinen M, Dietz R, Neuhaus KL, Jánosi A, Thorgeirsson G, Dunselman PH, Gullestad L, Kuch J, Herlitz J, Rickenbacher P, Ball S, Gottlieb S, Deedwania P. Effects of controlled-release metoprolol on total mortality, hospitalizations, and well-being in patients with heart failure: the Metoprolol CR/XL Randomized Intervention Trial in congestive heart failure (MERIT-HF). MERIT-HF Study Group. JAMA. 2000;283: 1295–302.
63. The Cardiac Insufficiency Bisoprolol Study II (CIBIS-II): a randomised trial. Lancet. 1999;353:9–13.
64. Packer M, Bristow MR, Cohn JN, Colucci WS, Fowler MB, Gilbert EM, Shusterman NH. The effect of carvedilol on morbidity and mortality in patients with chronic heart failure. U.S. Carvedilol Heart Failure Study Group. N Engl J Med. 1996;334:1349–55.
65. Flather MD, Shibata MC, Coats AJS, Van Veldhuisen DJ, Parkhomenko A, Borbola J, Cohen-Solal A, Dumitrascu D, Ferrari R, Lechat P, Soler-Soler J, Tavazzi L, Spinarova L, Toman

J, Böhm M, Anker SD, Thompson SG, Poole-Wilson PA, SENIORS Investigators. Randomized trial to determine the effect of nebivolol on mortality and cardiovascular hospital admission in elderly patients with heart failure (SENIORS). Eur Heart J. 2005;26:215–25.

66. Pepine CJ, Handberg EM, Cooper-DeHoff RM, Marks RG, Kowey P, Messerli FH, Mancia G, Cangiano JL, Garcia-Barreto D, Keltai M, Erdine S, Bristol HA, Kolb HR, Bakris GL, Cohen JD, Parmley WW, INVEST Investigators. A calcium antagonist vs a non-calcium antagonist hypertension treatment strategy for patients with coronary artery disease. The International Verapamil-Trandolapril Study (INVEST): a randomized controlled trial. JAMA. 2003;290:2805–16.

67. Poole-Wilson PA, Lubsen J, Kirwan B-A, van Dalen FJ, Wagener G, Danchin N, Just H, Fox KAA, Pocock SJ, Clayton TC, Motro M, Parker JD, Bourassa MG, Dart AM, Hildebrandt P, Hjalmarson A, Kragten JA, Molhoek GP, Otterstad J-E, Seabra-Gomes R, Soler-Soler J, Weber S, Coronary disease Trial Investigating Outcome with Nifedipine gastrointestinal therapeutic system investigators. Effect of long-acting nifedipine on mortality and cardiovascular morbidity in patients with stable angina requiring treatment (ACTION trial): randomised controlled trial. Lancet. 2004;364:849–57.

68. Frishman WH, Glasser S, Stone P, Deedwania PC, Johnson M, Fakouhi TD. Comparison of controlled-onset, extended-release verapamil with amlodipine and amlodipine plus atenolol on exercise performance and ambulatory ischemia in patients with chronic stable angina pectoris. Am J Cardiol. 1999;83:507–14.

69. Nissen SE, Tuzcu EM, Libby P, Thompson PD, Ghali M, Garza D, Berman L, Shi H, Buebendorf E, Topol EJ, CAMELOT Investigators. Effect of antihypertensive agents on cardiovascular events in patients with coronary disease and normal blood pressure: the CAMELOT study: a randomized controlled trial. JAMA. 2004;292:2217–25.

70. Döring G. Antianginal and anti-ischemic efficacy of nicorandil in comparison with isosorbide-5-mononitrate and isosorbide dinitrate: results from two multicenter, double-blind, randomized studies with stable coronary heart disease patients. J Cardiovasc Pharmacol. 1992;20 Suppl 3:S74–81.

71. Di Somma S, Liguori V, Petitto M, Carotenuto A, Bokor D, de Divitiis O, de Divitiis M. A double-blind comparison of nicorandil

and metoprolol in stable effort angina pectoris. Cardiovasc Drugs Ther. 1993;7:119–23.

72. The SWAN Study Group. Comparison of the antiischaemic and antianginal effects of nicorandil and amlodipine in patients with symptomatic stable angina pectoris: the SWAN study. Journal of Basic and Clinical Cardiology. 1999;2:213–7.

73. Guermonprez JL, Blin P, Peterlongo F. A double-blind comparison of the long-term efficacy of a potassium channel opener and a calcium antagonist in stable angina pectoris. Eur Heart J. 1993;14 Suppl B:30–4.

74. IONA Study Group. Effect of nicorandil on coronary events in patients with stable angina: the Impact Of Nicorandil in Angina (IONA) randomised trial. Lancet. 2002;359:1269–75.

75. Cavero I, Djellas Y, Guillon JM. Ischemic myocardial cell protection conferred by the opening of ATP-sensitive potassium channels. Cardiovasc Drugs Ther. 1995;9 Suppl 2:245–55.

76. Sekiya M, Sato M, Funada J, Ohtani T, Akutsu H, Watanabe K. Effects of the long-term administration of nicorandil on vascular endothelial function and the progression of arteriosclerosis. J Cardiovasc Pharmacol. 2005;46:63–7.

77. Serizawa K-I, Yogo K, Aizawa K, Tashiro Y, Takahari Y, Sekine K, Suzuki T, Ishizuka N, Ishida H. Paclitaxel-induced endothelial dysfunction in living rats is prevented by nicorandil via reduction of oxidative stress. J Pharmacol Sci. 2012;119:349–58.

78. Ishibashi Y, Takahashi N, Tokumaru A, Karino K, Sugamori T, Sakane T, Yoshitomi H, Sato H, Oyake N, Murakami Y, Shimada T. Effects of long-term nicorandil administration on endothelial function, inflammation, and oxidative stress in patients without coronary artery disease. J Cardiovasc Pharmacol. 2008;51:311–6.

79. Falase B, Easaw J, Youhana A. The role of nicorandil in the treatment of myocardial ischaemia. Expert Opin Pharmacother. 2001;2:845–56.

80. Kaski JC, Hayward C, Mahida S, Baker S, Khong T, Tamargo J, editors. Drugs in cardiology: a comprehensive guide to cardiovascular pharmacotherapy. Oxford: Oxford University Press; 2010.

81. Wagner G. Selected issues from an overview on nicorandil: tolerance, duration of action, and long-term efficacy. J Cardiovasc Pharmacol. 1992;20 Suppl 3:S86–92.

82. Kool MJ, Spek JJ, Struyker Boudier HA, Hoeks AP, Reneman RS, van Herwaarden RH, Van Bortel LM. Acute and subacute effects of nicorandil and isosorbide dinitrate on vessel wall properties of large arteries and hemodynamics in healthy volunteers. Cardiovasc Drugs Ther. 1995;9:331–7.

83. Roland E. Safety profile of an anti-anginal agent with potassium channel opening activity: an overview. Eur Heart J. 1993;14 Suppl B:48–52.

84. Tardif J-C, Ford I, Tendera M, Bourassa MG, Fox K, INITIATIVE Investigators. Efficacy of ivabradine, a new selective I(f) inhibitor, compared with atenolol in patients with chronic stable angina. Eur Heart J. 2005;26:2529–36.

85. Tardif J-C, Ponikowski P, Kahan T, ASSOCIATE Study Investigators. Efficacy of the I(f) current inhibitor ivabradine in patients with chronic stable angina receiving beta-blocker therapy: a 4-month, randomized, placebo-controlled trial. Eur Heart J. 2009;30:540–8.

86. Ruzyllo W, Tendera M, Ford I, Fox KM. Antianginal efficacy and safety of ivabradine compared with amlodipine in patients with stable effort angina pectoris: a 3-month randomised, double-blind, multicentre, noninferiority trial. Drugs. 2007;67:393–405.

87. Jedlickova L, Merkovska L, Jackova L, Janicko M, Fedacko J, Novakova B, Chmelarova A, Majernik J, Pella D. Effect of ivabradine on endothelial function in patients with stable angina pectoris: assessment with the Endo-PAT 2000 device. Adv Ther. 2015;32:962–70.

88. Fox K, Ford I, Steg PG, Tendera M, Robertson M, Ferrari R, BEAUTIFUL investigators. Heart rate as a prognostic risk factor in patients with coronary artery disease and left-ventricular systolic dysfunction (BEAUTIFUL): a subgroup analysis of a randomised controlled trial. Lancet. 2008;372:817–21.

89. Heusch G, Skyschally A, Gres P, van Caster P, Schilawa D, Schulz R. Improvement of regional myocardial blood flow and function and reduction of infarct size with ivabradine: protection beyond heart rate reduction. Eur Heart J. 2008;29:2265–75.

90. Werdan K, Ebelt H, Nuding S, Höpfner F, Hack G, Müller-Werdan U. Ivabradine in combination with beta-blocker improves symptoms and quality of life in patients with stable angina pectoris: results from the ADDITIONS study. Clin Res Cardiol. 2012;101:365–73.

91. Camici PG, Gloekler S, Levy BI, Skalidis E, Tagliamonte E, Vardas P, Heusch G. Ivabradine in chronic stable angina: effects by and beyond heart rate reduction. Int J Cardiol. 2016;215:1–6.

92. Colin P, Ghaleh B, Monnet X, Su J, Hittinger L, Giudicelli J-F, Berdeaux A. Contributions of heart rate and contractility to myocardial oxygen balance during exercise. Am J Physiol Heart Circ Physiol. 2003;284:H676–82.

93. Dillinger J-G, Maher V, Vitale C, Henry P, Logeart D, Manzo Silberman S, Allée G, Levy BI. Impact of ivabradine on central aortic blood pressure and myocardial perfusion in patients with stable coronary artery disease. Hypertension. 2015;66:1138–44.

94. Tagliamonte E, Cirillo T, Rigo F, Astarita C, Coppola A, Romano C, Capuano N. Ivabradine and bisoprolol on Doppler-derived coronary flow velocity eeserve in patients with stable coronary artery disease: beyond the heart rate. Adv Ther. 2015;32:757–67.

95. Skalidis EI, Hamilos MI, Chlouverakis G, Zacharis EA, Vardas PE. Ivabradine improves coronary flow reserve in patients with stable coronary artery disease. Atherosclerosis. 2011;215:160–5.

96. Gloekler S, Traupe T, Stoller M, Schild D, Steck H, Khattab A, Vogel R, Seiler C. The effect of heart rate reduction by ivabradine on collateral function in patients with chronic stable coronary artery disease. Heart. 2014;100:160–6.

97. Fox K, Ford I, Steg PG, Tendera M, Robertson M, Ferrari R, BEAUTIFUL Investigators. Relationship between ivabradine treatment and cardiovascular outcomes in patients with stable coronary artery disease and left ventricular systolic dysfunction with limiting angina: a subgroup analysis of the randomized, controlled BEAUTIFUL trial. Eur Heart J. 2009;30:2337–45.

98. Drouin A, Gendron M-E, Thorin E, Gillis M-A, Mahlberg-Gaudin F, Tardif J-C. Chronic heart rate reduction by ivabradine prevents endothelial dysfunction in dyslipidaemic mice. Br J Pharmacol. 2008;154:749–57.

99. Custodis F, Baumhäkel M, Schlimmer N, List F, Gensch C, Böhm M, Laufs U. Heart rate reduction by ivabradine reduces oxidative stress, improves endothelial function, and prevents atherosclerosis in apolipoprotein E-deficient mice. Circulation. 2008;117:2377–87.

100. Fox K, Ford I, Steg PG, Tendera M, Ferrari R, BEAUTIFUL Investigators. Ivabradine for patients with stable coronary artery disease and left-ventricular systolic dysfunction (BEAUTIFUL): a randomised, double-blind, placebo-controlled trial. Lancet. 2008;372:807–16.

101. Fox K, Ford I, Steg PG, Tardif J-C, Tendera M, Ferrari R. Ivabradine in stable coronary artery disease without clinical heart failure. N Engl J Med. 2014;371:1091–9.

102. Fox K, Ford I, Steg PG, Tardif J-C, Tendera M, Ferrari R. Bradycardia and atrial fibrillation in patients with stable coronary artery disease treated with ivabradine: an analysis from the SIGNIFY study. European Heart Journal (2015);36:3291–6.

103. Stanley WC, Lopaschuk GD, Hall JL, McCormack JG. Regulation of myocardial carbohydrate metabolism under normal and ischaemic conditions. Potential for pharmacological interventions. Cardiovasc Res. 1997;33:243–57.

104. Stanley WC, Recchia FA, Lopaschuk GD. Myocardial substrate metabolism in the normal and failing heart. Physiol Rev. 2005;85:1093–129.

105. Jaswal JS, Keung W, Wang W, Ussher JR, Lopaschuk GD. Targeting fatty acid and carbohydrate oxidation – a novel therapeutic intervention in the ischemic and failing heart. Biochim Biophys Acta. 1813;2011:1333–50.

106. Fillmore N, et al. Mitochondrial fatty acid oxidation alterations in heart failure, ischemic heart disease and diabetic cardiomyopathy. Br J Pharmacol. 2014;171:2080–90.

107. Kantor PF, Lucien A, Kozak R, Lopaschuk GD. The antianginal drug trimetazidine shifts cardiac energy metabolism from fatty acid oxidation to glucose oxidation by inhibiting mitochondrial long-chain 3-ketoacyl coenzyme A thiolase. Circ Res. 2000;86:580–8.

108. Blardi P, de Lalla A, Volpi L, Auteri A, Di Perri T. Increase of adenosine plasma levels after oral trimetazidine: a pharmacological preconditioning? Pharmacol Res. 2002;45:69–72.

109. Poloński L, Dec I, Wojnar R, Wilczek K. Trimetazidine limits the effects of myocardial ischaemia during percutaneous coronary angioplasty. Curr Med Res Opin. 2002;18:389–96.

110. Szwed H. Clinical benefits of trimetazidine in patients with recurrent angina. Coron Artery Dis. 2004;15 Suppl 1:S17–21.

111. Szwed H, Sadowski Z, Elikowski W, Koronkiewicz A, Mamcarz A, Orszulak W, Skibińska E, Szymczak K, Swiatek J, Winter M. Combination treatment in stable effort angina using trimetazidine and metoprolol: results of a randomized, double-blind, multicentre study (TRIMPOL II). TRIMetazidine in POLand. Eur Heart J. 2001;22:2267–74.

112. Chazov EI, Lepakchin VK, Zharova EA, Fitilev SB, Levin AM, Rumiantzeva EG, Fitileva TB. Trimetazidine in Angina Combination Therapy – the TACT study: trimetazidine versus conventional treatment in patients with stable angina pectoris

in a randomized, placebo-controlled, multicenter study. Am J Ther. 2005;12:35–42.

113. Michaelides AP, Spiropoulos K, Dimopoulos K, Athanasiades D, Toutouzas P. Antianginal efficacy of the combination of trimetazidine-propranolol compared with isosorbide dinitrate-propranolol in patients with stable angina. Clin Drug Investig. 1997;13:8–14.

114. Vitale C, Spoletini I, Malorni W, Perrone-Filardi P, Volterrani M, Rosano GMC. Efficacy of trimetazidine on functional capacity in symptomatic patients with stable exertional angina – the VASCO-angina study. Int J Cardiol. 2013;168:1078–81.

115. Danchin N, Marzilli M, Parkhomenko A, Ribeiro JP. Efficacy comparison of trimetazidine with therapeutic alternatives in stable angina pectoris: a network meta-analysis. Cardiology. 2011;120:59–72.

116. Chen J, Zhou S, Jin J, Tian F, Han Y, Wang J, Liu J, Chen Y. Chronic treatment with trimetazidine after discharge reduces the incidence of restenosis in patients who received coronary stent implantation: a 1-year prospective follow-up study. Int J Cardiol. 2014;174:634–9.

117. Yoon JW, Cho BJ, Park HS, Kang SM, Choi SH, Jang HC, Shin H, Lee MJ, Kim YB, Park KS, Lim S. Differential effects of trimetazidine on vascular smooth muscle cell and endothelial cell in response to carotid artery balloon injury in diabetic rats. Int J Cardiol. 2013;167:126–33.

118. Cole PL, Beamer AD, McGowan N, Cantillon CO, Benfell K, Kelly RA, Hartley LH, Smith TW, Antman EM. Efficacy and safety of perhexiline maleate in refractory angina. A double-blind placebo-controlled clinical trial of a novel antianginal agent. Circulation. 1990;81:1260–70.

119. Klassen GA, Zborowska-Sluis DT, Wright GJ. Effects of oral perhexiline on canine myocardial flow distribution. Can J Physiol Pharmacol. 1980;58:543–9.

120. Unger SA, Kennedy JA, McFadden-Lewis K, Minerds K, Murphy GA, Horowitz JD. Dissociation between metabolic and efficiency effects of perhexiline in normoxic rat myocardium. J Cardiovasc Pharmacol. 2005;46:849–55.

121. Barclay ML, Sawyers SM, Begg EJ, Zhang M, Roberts RL, Kennedy MA, Elliott JM. Correlation of CYP2D6 genotype with perhexiline phenotypic metabolizer status. Pharmacogenetics. 2003;13:627–32.

122. Reddy BM, Weintraub HS, Schwartzbard AZ. Ranolazine: a new approach to treating an old problem. Tex Heart Inst J. 2010;37:641–7.

123. Tarkin JM, Kaski JC. Pharmacological treatment of chronic stable angina pectoris. Clin Med. 2013;13:63–70.

124. Deshmukh SH, Patel SR, Pinassi E, Mindrescu C, Hermance EV, Infantino MN, Coppola JT, Staniloae CS. Ranolazine improves endothelial function in patients with stable coronary artery disease. Coron Artery Dis. 2009;20:343–7.

125. Chaitman BR, Skettino SL, Parker JO, Hanley P, Meluzin J, Kuch J, Pepine CJ, Wang W, Nelson JJ, Hebert DA, Wolff AA, MARISA Investigators. Anti-ischemic effects and long-term survival during ranolazine monotherapy in patients with chronic severe angina. J Am Coll Cardiol. 2004;43:1375–82.

126. Chaitman BR, Pepine CJ, Parker JO, Skopal J, Chumakova G, Kuch J, Wang W, Skettino SL, Wolff AA. Effects of ranolazine with atenolol, amlodipine, or diltiazem on exercise tolerance and angina frequency in patients with severe chronic angina: a randomized controlled trial. JAMA. 2004;291:309–16.

127. Stone PH, Gratsiansky NA, Blokhin A, Huang I-Z, Meng L, ERICA Investigators. Antianginal efficacy of ranolazine when added to treatment with amlodipine: the ERICA (Efficacy of Ranolazine in Chronic Angina) trial. J Am Coll Cardiol. 2006;48:566–75.

128. Kosiborod M, Arnold SV, Spertus JA, McGuire DK, Li Y, Yue P, Ben-Yehuda O, Katz A, Jones PG, Olmsted A, Belardinelli L, Chaitman BR. Evaluation of ranolazine in patients with type 2 diabetes mellitus and chronic stable angina: results from the TERISA randomized clinical trial (Type 2 Diabetes Evaluation of Ranolazine in Subjects With Chronic Stable Angina). J Am Coll Cardiol. 2013;61:2038–45.

129. Alexander KP, Weisz G, Prather K, James S, Mark DB, Anstrom KJ, Davidson-Ray L, Witkowski A, Mulkay AJ, Osmukhina A, Farzaneh-Far R, Ben-Yehuda O, Stone GW, Ohman EM. Effects of ranolazine on angina and quality of life after percutaneous coronary intervention with incomplete revascularization: results from the ranolazine for incomplete vessel revascularization (RIVER-PCI) trial. Circulation. 2016;133:39–47.

130. Morrow DA, Scirica BM, Karwatowska-Prokopczuk E, Murphy SA, Budaj A, Varshavsky S, Wolff AA, Skene A, McCabe CH, Braunwald E, MERLIN-TIMI 36 Trial Investigators. Effects of ranolazine on recurrent cardiovascu-

lar events in patients with non-ST-elevation acute coronary syndromes: the MERLIN-TIMI 36 randomized trial. JAMA. 2007;297:1775–83.

131. Noman A, Ang DSC, Ogston S, Lang CC, Struthers AD. Effect of high-dose allopurinol on exercise in patients with chronic stable angina: a randomised, placebo controlled crossover trial. Lancet. 2010;375:2161–7.

132. Christian TF, Miller TD, Bailey KR, Gibbons RJ. Exercise tomographic thallium-201 imaging in patients with severe coronary artery disease and normal electrocardiograms. Ann Intern Med. 1994;121:825–32.

133. Wagner F, Gohlke-Bärwolf C, Trenk D, Jähnchen E, Roskamm H. Differences in the antiischaemic effects of molsidomine and isosorbide dinitrate (ISDN) during acute and short-term administration in stable angina pectoris. Eur Heart J. 1991;12:994–9.

134. Piccolo R, Giustino G, Mehran R, Windecker S. Stable coronary artery disease: revascularisation and invasive strategies. Lancet. 2015;386:702–13.

135. Windecker S, Stortecky S, Stefanini GG, da Costa BR, Rutjes AW, Di Nisio M, Silletta MG, Siletta MG, Maione A, Alfonso F, Clemmensen PM, Collet J-P, Cremer J, Falk V, Filippatos G, Hamm C, Head S, Kappetein AP, Kastrati A, Knuuti J, Landmesser U, Laufer G, Neumann F-J, Richter D, Schauerte P, Sousa Uva M, Taggart DP, Torracca L, Valgimigli M, et al. Revascularisation versus medical treatment in patients with stable coronary artery disease: network meta-analysis. BMJ. 2014;348:g3859.

136. Boden WE, O'Rourke RA, Teo KK, Hartigan PM, Maron DJ, Kostuk WJ, Knudtson M, Dada M, Casperson P, Harris CL, Chaitman BR, Shaw L, Gosselin G, Nawaz S, Title LM, Gau G, Blaustein AS, Booth DC, Bates ER, Spertus JA, Berman DS, Mancini GBJ, Weintraub WS, COURAGE Trial Research Group. Optimal medical therapy with or without PCI for stable coronary disease. N Engl J Med. 2007;356:1503–16.

137. Johnson NP, Tóth GG, Lai D, Zhu H, Açar G, Agostoni P, Appelman Y, Arslan F, Barbato E, Chen S-L, Di Serafino L, Domínguez-Franco AJ, Dupouy P, Esen AM, Esen OB, Hamilos M, Iwasaki K, Jensen LO, Jiménez-Navarro MF, Katritsis DG, Kocaman SA, Koo B-K, López-Palop R, Lorin JD, Miller LH, Muller O, Nam C-W, Oud N, Puymirat E, Rieber J, et al. Prognostic value of fractional flow reserve: linking physiologic severity to clinical outcomes. J Am Coll Cardiol. 2014;64:1641–54.

138. Leape LL, Park RE, Bashore TM, Harrison JK, Davidson CJ, Brook RH. Effect of variability in the interpretation of coronary angiograms on the appropriateness of use of coronary revascularization procedures. Am Heart J. 2000;139:106–13.

139. Takaro T, Hultgren HN, Lipton MJ, Detre KM. The VA cooperative randomized study of surgery for coronary arterial occlusive disease II. Subgroup with significant left main lesions. Circulation. 1976;54:III107–17.

140. Takaro T, Hultgren HN, Detre KM, Peduzzi P. The Veterans Administration Cooperative Study of stable angina: current status. Circulation. 1982;65:60–7.

141. Yusuf S, Zucker D, Peduzzi P, Fisher LD, Takaro T, Kennedy JW, Davis K, Killip T, Passamani E, Norris R. Effect of coronary artery bypass graft surgery on survival: overview of 10-year results from randomised trials by the Coronary Artery Bypass Graft Surgery Trialists Collaboration. Lancet. 1994;344:563–70.

142. Taylor HA, Deumite NJ, Chaitman BR, Davis KB, Killip T, Rogers WJ. Asymptomatic left main coronary artery disease in the Coronary Artery Surgery Study (CASS) registry. Circulation. 1989;79:1171–9.

143. Caracciolo EA, Davis KB, Sopko G, Kaiser GC, Corley SD, Schaff H, Taylor HA, Chaitman BR. Comparison of surgical and medical group survival in patients with left main equivalent coronary artery disease. Long-term CASS experience. Circulation. 1995;91:2335–44.